THE
BOOK
OF THE
PENIS

THE
BOOK
OF THE
PENIS

Maggie
Paley

Illustrations by Sergio Ruzzier

Grove Press

Published simultaneously in Canada
Printed in the United States of America

FIRST EDITION

Library of Congress Cataloging-in-Publication Data

Paley, Maggie.
    The book of the penis / Maggie Paley ; illustrations by Sergio
Ruzzier.
        p.   cm.
    Includes bibliographical references.
    ISBN 0-8021-1648-5
    1. Penis—History.   2. Penis—Social aspects.   I. Title.
GT498.P45P35   1999
573.6'56—dc21   99-20348
                                                                CIP

Design by Charles Rue Woods

Grove Press
841 Broadway
New York, NY 10003

99 00 01 02   10 9 8 7 6 5 4 3 2 1

CONTENTS

CONTENTS

CONTENTS

CONTENTS

PREFACE

Until recently, few people used penis, the word, in conversation. It seemed, somehow, too naked. At least slang expressions had a comradely feeling. Dick, cock, prick, pecker—they were things you could whisper with affection, or growl with affectionate disdain, or use to curse with. Then in 1993 John Wayne Bobbitt, a small-town Southern ex-Marine, had his penis lopped off by his wife and sewn back on, and the story was so sensational that the word was all over the news. The *New York Times*, which had used it only three times in the preceding twenty years, was printing it every day. Late-night talk-show hosts began to make jokes—first about Bobbitt's penis, then about penises in general. Slowly the word spread, until it was even coming up in small talk, with people you hardly knew. The speaker who used it always got credit for frankness—but the word still made most people wince. After all, in the West, at least, we were brought up to pretend the penis wasn't there.

Since I first started working on this book I've had countless conversations about penises, all of them somewhat embarrassing. In the first place, once the penis comes up, almost anything you say becomes a double entendre. So many simple basic words are penis-related: in, out, hard, soft, head, tail and so on. I was also embarrassed by the unspoken question I often felt hovering in the air. It was the question my father would have asked had he still been alive: What went wrong, darling? Aren't you a lady anymore?

The first time I remember seeing a penis I was maybe ten years old, taking the subway home from school by myself. While I was waiting for the train, a man down the platform took his penis out of his pants and showed it to me. He was a black man. I was so intent on not noticing any such thing that at first I imagined he was offering me a chocolate-covered candy bar. I knew just enough to turn the other way and find a nice older woman to stand next to, pretending she was my mother.

About five years later it happened again. I was with my first grown-up boyfriend, a college senior. We were necking one evening in the front seat of his parked car and he took his penis out of his pants and showed it to me. Oh, no, I said to myself. Is this what I'm going to have to put up with if I want to be a woman and have sex? Because it was as ugly as a monster from outer space, and it seemed to have him in its power. He was obviously more interested in it than he was in me. He'd taken it out so I would kiss it and make it feel better. It looked so unreasonable, thrusting forward, veins bulging, head inflamed, as if it wanted to move, to leave the front seat of the car and go find something cool to plunge itself into, dragging the boyfriend behind.

"You want me to do what?" I said.

"Just kiss it," he said. "Please."

Some women say they don't like penises, preferring buttocks and shoulders. But really, what good is a shoulder going to do you?

Sensing where my interests lay, I got used to the penis —not that boy's, but someone else's, and someone else's after that—and I began to feel its power and see its beauty and even to admire its persistence. Because a penis with a passion is capable of almost anything, isn't it? Yet I never asked questions about it and never examined one too closely. I thought it would be impolite to stare.

In any case there was no way I could ask what I really wanted to know—which was what did it feel like to have one. If I knew that, I believed, I would understand men, and I wouldn't get impatient with their weird penis-inspired behavior.

Then, inevitably, I met Enrique, a man who liked to talk about the penis. He had been an altar boy, growing up in Caracas. He had loved the Church, and also loved his penis. He couldn't understand why the Church said touching his penis was bad. So he had read up on the penis, and in the end he had left the Church.

Over dinner Enrique would speak of Henry VIII's armor, which he said was in the tower of London and had an enormous protruding codpiece. He would discuss penis enlargement surgery, and techniques for prolonging erection and having multiple orgasms. He would mention the Mayan kings who ritually pierced their penises with sting-ray spines or awls made of animal bone, so their blood could fertilize the land. He would talk of the seven-foot phalluses paraded by Shinto priests through the streets of Japan. "It is beautiful, and so touching, isn't it?" he would say, and he would smile a dreamy smile.

I began to see there was a penis culture that existed in the midst of regular culture, exerting its influence though almost no one spoke of it, at least not to me. "That's very interesting," I said to Enrique.

"Write a book about it," Enrique said.

It would be too embarrassing being the author of such a book. I didn't even want to think about it. And yet I couldn't stop thinking about it; the idea hung around until in the end I decided embarrassment might be good for me.

So I set out to explore the territory—and as soon as I did my life started to change. I became popular in ways I could never have imagined. Every party I went to, a friend would mention that I was writing a book about penises, and then there would be people who had penis stories and penis questions and nobody would talk to me about anything else. Men showed a new interest, and I wasn't sure it was the kind of interest I wanted. At home I pored over dirty books. Three different people gave me boxes of penis pasta for Christmas. I persevered, hoping to reach some natural conclusions. The conclusion I came to, after a year of reading, interviewing and visiting phallic places, was that this was one enormous subject.

I've only managed to skim the surface of the subject, and I leave it to someone else to plumb its depths. What you have in your hands is an explorer's book, partly an account of where I went and what I heard and saw, partly a recounting of the information I uncovered.

First, a few general observations:

Riddle: Why do so many men have names for their dicks?

Answer: Would you want to be bossed around by somebody you don't even know?

The most obvious difference between men and women is that men have protruding sex organs. Every time a man looks down, there's his penis—his little friend. Women don't feel the same friendship for their vaginas or vulvas, no doubt because it takes such an effort to see them. It's hard to become pals with something you can't see. But men are fascinated by their penises, and who wouldn't be? A penis, though it's part of a man, clearly shows signs of being a separate entity. Penises change size, shape and color as if by magic. Small as they are in relation to body size, they lead enormous men around. One man informed me he calls his penis "companion of my finest hours." No one tells women this, but a man's relationship with his penis may be the most important relationship in his life.

Otherwise, why would men have built a penis-centered world, full of things that look like penises or work in the way penises work. Penis-looking things are usually men's things—guns, cars, rockets, cigars, skyscrapers. Men are comfortable around them and see them as power symbols, just as penises are power symbols.

It can't be easy, being a man. The minute you have a penis, you're in competition with all the other penises, vying for fucking rights. Not only that, you worry about losing it. Freud believed that this worry, which he called castration anxiety, was at the root of the trouble between men and women: Men are afraid of women because they're afraid of *becoming* women—dickless people.

Freud, who was perhaps a bit penis-obsessed, also thought women suffered from penis envy, wanting dicks of their own. One reason his theories are not as influential as they used to be is that for all his genius he couldn't know how women felt about penises. Few adult women would actually want a big slippery penis attached to their bodies, though they might want the power that goes with having one. As a number of writers have already pointed out, penis envy is more a male phenomenon.

Of course, the reason we care so much about penises is that they have erections. Without erections a penis would be just a urination device, a thing without allure. Erect, a penis is a sex machine. An erect penis is a reminder of the miraculous transformation it has just been through and of the act it was created to perform—ejaculating sperm in order to make new life, or "sharing its load," as the advertisements for phone sex on direct access cable would have it. Every man wants to have the biggest erection in town, and he's envious of other men who might outdo him.

Over the course of a year I asked a number of men to talk to me about their relationships with their penises. My aim was to find out what penises mean to men, and how this affects their relationship with the world, with each other and with women. All my informants were volunteers. Long before I got the tape recorder out, most of the heterosexual men had offered to show it to me. On the other hand, they didn't have all that much to say about it. Either they didn't know how to say it, or they didn't want to say it and be embarrassed. The gay men I interviewed knew more about the subject, and were more forthcoming. But even most of them were shy. One, the composer Ned Rorem, told me later that he would have said things to a male interviewer that he couldn't bring himself to say to a woman.

When it comes to their dicks, men can't behave rationally. They love them, but they're embarrassed about the things they do or want to do with them—masturbate, get a blow job, penetrate someone in every orifice, whatever. Even if they just want to make tender love they're likely to be embarrassed because feelings tend to embarrass men. Yet, inspired by their penises, men will go to extraordinary, extravagant, outrageous extremes. I've noted those extremes wherever I've found them.

My object is to open this subject up for you, so you can smile when you think about it.

PART

ONE

THE NATURE

OF PENISES

*T*his section is about the physical nature of penises, and it brings up some interesting questions.

What causes an erection? Does size matter? What size is average? Can you tell a man's penis size by the size of his hands or feet? Is penis enlargement surgery worth the risk? Can you stretch your penis with weights? Do big dicks have more fun?

To get some answers, read on.

CHAPTER ONE

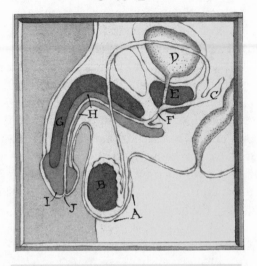

A SCROTUM
B TESTICLE (ONE OF A PAIR)
C SEMINAL VESICLE (ONE OF A PAIR)
D BLADDER
E PROSTATE GLAND
F URETHRA
G CORPUS CAVERNOSUM (ONE OF A PAIR)
H CORPUS SPONGIOSUM
I HEAD (GLANS)
J URETHRA OPENING

PENIS
PHYSIOLOGY

Penis size and shape are hereditary, and penises are as similar on the whole as they are infinite in their variety. They are not muscles, and there's no bone in any of them.

THE NATURE OF PENISES

The penis is attached to the pelvic cavity at its root, or base. Its head, the big, smooth cap on the end, is called the glans, and the rim around the base of the glans is the corona. The shaft of the penis contains three columns of spongy erectile tissue, and is encased in a loose layer of skin. In uncircumcised men this skin also covers the glans. The piece of skin that keeps the glans covered is known as the foreskin, or prepuce, and it retracts as the penis becomes erect. Circumcised men have had the foreskin removed, so that the head of the penis is uncovered at all times. The slit in the head is the opening of the urethra, a slim tube that runs from the bladder through the body of the penis to the head. The urethra carries both urine and semen to the outside world, but not simultaneously.

The penis rests on the scrotum, which contains two testicles, or balls. Both testosterone and sperm are manufactured in the testicles.

Penis and testicles grow to full size during puberty. From puberty onward, the sperm factory in the testicles maintains a constant production cycle. A healthy, fertile male makes several hundred million tiny sperm each day. His penis functions as a conveyor belt. Its erection is a sign he's getting ready to discharge some of those sperm, depositing them perhaps with a fellow human and in any case clearing his own storage facility for further stockpiling.

ERECTIONS

No one knows why men have erections when they have them and not when they don't. Clearly they happen in response to erotic stimulation, but this stimulation can be purely physical or purely inspired by the imagination and the senses other than touch, or some combination of the two. Ned Rorem, in his memoir, *Knowing When to Stop,* reports what he was told about the French poet and film-maker Jean Cocteau, "that, as a parlor trick, [he] used to lie naked on his back, and surrounded by a cheering section, with no manipulation, no friction of any kind, would achieve ejaculation. . . ."

Though men have erections when they're sexually excited, they also have them when presumably they're not. Teenage boys have erections when they least expect them. Fear can also cause erections. And a man can desire sex and be so tense, for whatever reason, that his erection doesn't materialize. Or, especially when he gets older, he may be thwarted by physical problems.

One seventy-year-old man told me he couldn't count on his penis to get erections anymore. "In youth and middle age having a penis can be a source of enthusiasm for the world and for expressing oneself to others," he said. "I no longer always like having a penis."

A sure sign of the high value we place on erections is the word we use to describe a man who's unable to have or sustain an erection. We call him impotent, which means without power. Even though we now have a politically correct euphemism for impotence, erectile dysfunction, everyone knows exactly what that means.

Temporary impotence happens to every man some-times, and it's always a big embarrassment. The more a man worries about it, the more likely it is to happen again. If it begins to happen most of the time the impotence is in all probability no longer temporary—and according to figures released when the first erection pill, Viagra, went on the market in April of 1998, some 30 million American men are in this category. Yet in 1997, for example, only 2.6 million saw their doctors to try to do something about it—and of those only 628,000 were new patients.

In 1998 urologists became the nation's busiest doctors, working day and night writing out Viagra prescriptions. But before the advent of Viagra—which is said to solve the problem for 60 to 80 percent of those men who take it—impotence was not the sort of thing men liked to acknowledge by talking about it. For that reason little attention was paid to it by the medical profession in spite of the fact that most doctors are men, and it wasn't until the 1970s that the physiology of an erection was fully understood.

(Altogether, we people are awfully slow about understanding our bodies. Homo sapiens were a fully developed species, having sex with each other for some hundred thousand years, before we figured out where babies came from. Until the Neolithic period, around 9000 B.C., no one knew men had anything to do with conception. As soon as men realized what their role must be, presumably from studying animals, they began to lord it over women.)

PHYSIOLOGY OF AN ERECTION

When a man is sexually excited, the chemicals he secretes allow extra blood to be pumped into the erectile tissue of his penis. At the same time the erection itself presses on the veins, reducing outflow. An erect penis is a penis engorged with blood. Which is why the comic Robin Williams once said, "God gave us all a penis and a brain, but only enough blood to run one at a time."

Penises grow erect from base to head. One man described the feeling to me—"There's a faint warmth and sense of well-being, as if the sun has just moved over and covered you." The angle of erection varies from man to man but in general the younger a man is, the more his erections point up. As a man gets older he takes longer to reach a full erection and he may need direct stimulation of his penis.

During sex a man's testicles also increase in size and in most men at a certain point they elevate, pressing up against the pelvis. This elevation means ejaculation is near.

Ejaculation happens in two stages. Semen is formed during the first stage, when rhythmic contractions propel sperm from the testicles into the urethra to mix with seminal fluid from the seminal vesicles and the prostate. A man who experiences these contractions may say, "I'm coming"; he feels he's on the verge of orgasm, and at the point of no return.

During the second stage of ejaculation, contractions of the urethra, the prostate and the pelvic muscles propel the semen out the opening of the urethra. About a teaspoonful, containing 100 to 600 million sperm, is ejaculated at one time.

Here in the West we assume that orgasm, the intensely pleasurable feeling that accompanies ejaculation, can only occur during ejaculation—but this is not the case. Ejaculation is possible without orgasm (boys do it when they have wet dreams), and orgasm is possible without ejaculation. According to Chinese and Indian philosophies, orgasm without ejaculation is the path to ecstasy and superior health.

Orgasm can feel localized in the penis and testicles, or it can be more of a whole body experience. In the *Hite Report on Male Sexuality* one man says the sensation travels "down the back of my legs to the knees, up around my

7

arms into my deep insides. The penis is only the focus for all this, the trigger." Another says, "I feel like my cock has roots that extend down the backs of my legs, and coming draws juice from clear down there."

After ejaculation the erection subsides, either at once or gradually, and for a short time a man's penis and balls may be very tender.

If a man becomes highly excited and doesn't ejaculate, his erection takes longer to go away and he may feel a heaviness and discomfort in his testicles. However, this condition, known as "blue balls," is not at all as painful as teenage boys, trying to seduce teenage girls, like to claim it is.

THINKING WITH YOUR DICK

According to Darwinians—who use the theory of evolution to explain our behavior—humans are designed to be part monogamous, part promiscuous: The war between the sexes is more or less built into our biology. Men are nature's vehicles of sperm distribution—and they amass power in order to obtain sexual access for themselves. Sultans with harems, rich men with wives and mistresses, are merely following a biological imperative to reproduce. But women, the ones who have the babies, need to be choosier about their mates—they demand fidelity so that their young will be well fed and taken care of.

One gay man described to me what "thinking with your dick" means. "When you're stimulated, you switch into a different mode, and your dick takes over. It's a little like a horse that gets the bit in his mouth and runs. I'm talking about a completely physiological kind of thing.

That's why male/male sexuality is so combustible—you've got two combustible elements. There's a lot of sex in semi-public places like men's rooms and bars. They're there, they feel like it and they do it."

If this theory is correct then women, with our insistence on decorum, are the only obstacle standing between current courtship practices and a continuous, semipublic, erotic free-for-all.

CHAPTER

TWO

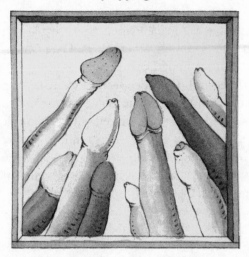

THE SIZE
QUESTION

Most men know what size penis they have because they've measured their erections. Some are happy with their size, but the majority would rather be bigger. Some of those who are not happy are actually bigger than average—they feel small anyway. To all men a big dick seems to be somewhat magical—much as beauty seems to be in women. Just as certain women may yearn for beauty and believe that if they had it their lives would be transformed, so do certain men yearn for longer, wider penises.

Even those men who are happy with their size begin to bristle when you talk to them about somebody *really* well endowed. Long Dong Silver, for example. Long Dong Silver is the porn star who became world-famous, briefly, when he was mentioned during the 1991 confirmation

THE NATURE OF PENISES

hearings for Supreme Court Justice Clarence Thomas. Anita Hill, as a character witness against Judge Thomas, said the judge had made inappropriate sexual remarks to her concerning, among other things, Long Dong.

You can see Long Dong in a video called *Long Dong Silver: The Legend*. The video seems to have been made up of odd bits and pieces; there isn't even the pretense of a story, and Long Dong is on-screen only sporadically—but you keeping watching, waiting for him to appear again. He's a nice-looking black man with well-developed buttock muscles and an eighteen-inch, knee-length penis. One of his tricks is to tilt his pelvis so that his penis swings from side to side like a wobbly pendulum. "Is that erect, or not?" men always ask. Who knows? It seems to be extended at all times, but it points down, not up. If it pointed up it would reach as high as his heart; if it pointed straight out you could hang laundry on it. Maybe it points out or up when he has sex. There are a few scenes of Long Dong having sex in the video, but they're shot from behind so you can't see what his dong is doing. You can see the face of the woman he's engaged with and she appears to be in agony. On the sound track is the Long Dong Silver song—a jaunty ballad about the man and his adventures with "what hangs between his knees."

In fact, a huge penis may not be altogether an asset. Franklin Russell, the naturalist writer, told me he had a friend who had a really outsized penis. "You realize," Russell said, "that an erection is a vascular event. The blood rushes to the penis. This huge guy confided in me. He said, 'I don't dare get a hard-on. I'm afraid I'll black out.'"

Vatsyayana, author of the *Kama Sutra*, divided men into three classes according to penis size: the hare, the bull and the horse. He also classified women by the size of their vaginas, as deer, mares and elephants. And he made the

12

sensible observation that the most comfortable sexual unions are between equals—the hare man with the deer woman, the bull man with the mare woman, the horse man with the elephant woman. The same is no doubt true today, and yet to men it seems to be beside the point.

WHAT'S WRONG WITH SMALL?

Women are small and feminine, men are big and masculine. A man's penis is the visible evidence of his virility. Penises are also the ultimate power symbols—but that's big, erect penises. No one builds an important building, or a rocket, in the shape of a limp little dick.

To see a penis enlarge and stiffen is to witness a miracle of nature; it's like watching time-lapse photography of a week in the life of a vegetable—seeing it go from wilted flower to big zucchini in a matter of moments. If that happens all the time, on your own body, you can't be blamed for concluding bigger is better. Especially because an erection alters a man. In the rest of his life he may be successful or ambitious or a layabout, but once he has an erection he's a man with a powerful purpose. Nature is using him to sow some seed.

Most of the time it's clear that size is an advantage. If you have more money or more land you have more ease and also more power. Big creatures have more physical strength than small ones. Big muscles are more powerful, long legs can run faster. An army has a better chance of winning than would one man fighting alone. The fate that rules our lives is so much bigger than we are that it surrounds us on all sides and we can't do anything about it.

13

HOW BIG IS BIG?

Women think of penis size as a sensitive issue. We're trained that way. I did not, for example, ask any of the men I interviewed what size they were because I felt it would be violating a trust. In fact I had never thought of penises in terms of inches before. Whatever man I was with, if he really wanted me to I would tell him he had the biggest cock I'd ever seen. I didn't think facts were the point, and for this reason I expected statistics about size to be hard to find.

To the contrary, the penis size of the American man has been well documented. Anyone who wants can look up the ongoing Definitive Penis Size Survey, a popular web site on the Internet. The results of this survey, which are periodically updated, are almost identical with the results obtained by Alfred Kinsey, who did his research on college men in the 1930s and '40s.

Very few American men are more than 9 inches long when erect, and very few are officially undersized. (At a web site advertising penis enlargement surgery the potential customer is informed that such surgery is considered to be cosmetic unless a man has a certifiable micropenis. If his erect penis is less than $3^{2}/_{3}$ inches long and less than $3\frac{1}{2}$ inches in circumference when erect, he may have surgery to lengthen his penis, and most likely his health insurance will cover it.) Most men—about 80 percent—measure between 5 and 7 inches erect. The greatest number are 6 to $6\frac{1}{2}$ inches long. Most men have a circumference, when erect, of between $4\frac{1}{2}$ and $5\frac{1}{2}$ inches.

But who wants to be average? Kurt Vonnegut told me that when his novel *Breakfast of Champions* was published the people at West Point gave him a hard time. In the middle of the book he had divulged the penis sizes of some of the male characters. Among them was a career army officer: "He had a penis six and one-half inches long and one and seven-eighths inches in diameter." The army felt he should have been bigger.

One of my informants said he used to play baseball in college, and he and his teammates would make comparisons, saying, "Whose is longer?" Meaning, he said, who has more character, heart and guts.

Since in cultures such as ours penis size is every man's secret, people like to guess how big a man is by looking at him. Folk wisdom has it you can tell a man's penis size from the size of his feet, or his hands, or his fingers, or his nose. Once I saw, passed around on a late-night talk show on TV, the basketball shoe of a seven-foot pro. The shoe was bigger than a baby, and everyone who saw it must have been visualizing the penis that went with it. But so far there haven't been any conclusive statistical studies. Anecdotal evidence suggests that hand and foot size may have some relationship to penis size. Noses, no.

Penises are unpredictable. You can't tell from the size of a flaccid penis what it will look like when it's erect. Some of those that look biggest when flaccid enlarge the least upon erection. One popular myth is that black men have the kind that enlarge the least, and the only reason white men think black men have bigger penises is that they see them in the locker room when they're limp. There are various other unconfirmed rumors about ethnic groups: that Arabs are particularly well hung, or that Latinos are. Jamaicans, I was told, are famously huge. They advertise in the gay porn magazine personal ads—you see them one after another: Jamaican, 10 inches; Jamaican, 11 inches. A male hustler I interviewed said eastern Europeans were biggest of all. These rumors are titillating. Anyone who's never thought of having sex with a Jamaican man can think about it now. Dreadlocks, that wonderful, lilting accent and a ten-inch wong.

According to two surprising news items that were posted on the Internet, in 1992 a World Health Organization survey found that more than a third of British penises were too big for their own government-approved condoms. A dispute was raging because the same British dicks were said to be bigger than the condom norm—17cm (about 6.7 inches) length and 5.6cm (about 2.2 inches) width— proposed for adoption by the European Economic Community.

That black men are bigger than white men, and that Asian men are smaller, are the two most popular racial stereotypes. Ned Rorem, who has written openly about his gay love life, challenges these stereotypes. "Whenever a race is called inferior, the men are said to have big dicks. All homosexuals have big dicks. All black men have big dicks. All Asians have small dicks. But the few Asians I've had any dealings with had perfectly normal-size dicks," he said to me. It's a point well taken. But many others I spoke with who were in a position to know—some gay men, a few adventurous women, a urologist—said black men *are* bigger and Asian men *are* smaller. (Since there is no hard scientific evidence, it's safe to conclude that your chance of getting the size you want, with any particular man, is about the same as your chance of having a coin you flip come up heads.)

Gay men also say that the most feminine among them often have big penises under their pants or skirts. The irony of course is that a big penis is supposed to be ultra-masculine. But no man you told about fabulously well endowed drag queens would come to the obvious conclusion that penis size might not be a measure of masculinity. The belief goes far too deep and may even be wired into male brains.

DICKS ON DISPLAY

After all, humans are basically a form of ape. We don't have thick, matted body hair, and we speak many languages and fly ourselves to Mars, but when it comes to sexuality we're in the same category as chimps and orangutans. We're not exactly the same as they are—because for one thing our males have much bigger penises in relation to body size. Darwinians, always on the lookout for nature's intention, believe human penises got big because they were being used for purposes of display. In other words, when a man pulls it out and shows it off, he's just doing what comes naturally.

Jared Diamond, in a charming article in *Discover* in 1996, compared the human penis to the sixteen-inch tail of the male long-tailed widowbird and the black stripe on the breast of another bird, the great tit. Female widowbirds are attracted to the males with the longest tails. Male great tits with wide black stripes on their breasts automatically dominate male great tits whose black stripes are not so wide. In the same way, he says, the human penis must have been seen as a sign of virility: The bigger a man's penis was, the more attractive he was to women and the more he was respected and feared by other men. If men had their way they would have penises as big as scimitars, or baseball bats, or cannons, with which they could really intimidate each other. Luckily, natural "counterselection" has kept their size within bounds. In evolutionary terms, a penis loses its rationale if it can't fit inside a vagina.

(Darwinians use comparative ball size among the great apes to prove that human reproductive strategy is meant to be mixed. Humans have medium-size balls, bigger than gorilla balls, smaller than chimps'. Small-balled gorillas hardly ever have sex, and they live in small bands with one male ruling several females, unchallenged by other males. Under these conditions they don't need much sperm in order to propagate. Chimps need big balls because they're promiscuous. The males who produce the most sperm have the best chance of impregnating females. Men's medium-size balls are ideally suited to a mixture of monogamy and promiscuity. Men need enough sperm to compete with other men, but the competition is limited.)

All their lives men see each other's flaccid dicks in locker rooms and at urinals. If it's true these dicks are fashioned for display, then how can the men help making comparisons? They look across at other men and down at themselves. Looking down has a foreshortening effect, so if they're the same size as everyone else, to themselves they look smaller.

Boys' penises start growing when they're about eleven, and stop when they're about seventeen. In high school the size competition is fiercest. Boys may get nicknames based on what their penises look like: the snake, the toad, the purple creeper. "You look at people's cocks when you take a shower in high school," I was told. "A guy with a good one shows it off. He'll flash it and wiggle it if he's with his friends in the same shower room—'How do you like this, huh?'"

Then before you know it boys become men, and they start considering penis enlargement surgery.

SMALL, ETC.

Small, Etc. is a club for men who are self-conscious about their penis size. Some really are small, according to "J," who founded the club in 1986. Most fall within the normal range, but feel small. Through the quarterly club magazine, *Small Gazette: The Smaller Man's Forum*, the six hundred members can communicate with each other and with J. *Small Gazette* publishes letters to the editor, the editor's advice, articles and sexual stories in which having a small penis turns out to be a plus. The bulk of the magazine, though, is devoted to personal ads—small men who want to correspond with others; gay and bisexual men who feel small, looking for lovers; and men of all sizes who are looking for small men to love.

J started the club "because I was self-conscious over my size and I felt there had to be other people out there who had experiences with rejection similar to mine."

I spoke with him on the phone.

Q: What kind of advice do you give other people who feel small?

A: Many people write, for instance, to ask if I have information about the operation to extend the size of the penis or to enhance the girth. I'll write to them and say that from everything I've been able to gather it's worse afterward; there are many side effects that are not revealed in the ads for penis extension, and many of the doctors performing the surgery are being sued. I'll tell them that increasing their self-esteem is really the key to feeling good about their size.

Q: What other questions are you most often asked?

A: I get letters from married men who feel they don't satisfy their wives. I get men who won't shower at the gym because they're afraid of what others might think of them. I get men who think they're bisexual but feel they don't measure up and other men won't be attracted to them. I get people who are afraid to have any sexual relationships because they fear they'll be humiliated, and they won't be able to give the other person what they anticipate they'll want.

THE NATURE OF PENISES

I get men in the club who are black, and people assume black men are very well endowed, and these men are not, they're just ordinary, and people say, What happened?

Q: How do you answer these people?

A: I tell them that I felt many of the fears and anxieties that they feel, and that my life has changed because I've been able to connect with others who also are small. Sometimes relating to people and knowing there are others out there like you can change your whole world.

Q: Do club members write to you about penis enlargement techniques other than surgery?

A: There are members who have had tremendous success with the penis pump, although most of the handheld ones don't really work. And it only helps temporarily, unless you use it over years and years and years.

Q: What about weights?

A: I hear there's an organization that's into weights. They get together and talk, nude, with these weights attached.

Q: Any other enlargement methods?

A: They have pants and different items you can buy to give you the illusion of being well endowed. In fact you're not, but the idea is that people will think that you are. I used to wear them, that's how I know, and I did get a lot of people attracted to me because of the way they made me look. Of course, I had to make sure I didn't go that next step and let anyone see me undressed.

Q: Is the club just for gay men?

A: It's for anyone who feels small. A few years ago *Penthouse* did a story on us, and I heard from a lot of heterosexual men who felt inferior about their size and wanted to meet women. I tried to find some women who might be interested in them, but the women didn't respond, even though I offered them free membership. Some of the men joined anyway. They might just have wanted to correspond with somebody else who was small. Or they might have wanted to read the magazines and know there are others out there and not do anything besides that.

I met my lover through the club. He's short in stature, and he said to me, "You're so concerned about your penis size, but people who are short in stature also have a problem in this world. When they go to bars people pat them on the head. It's harder for them to get ahead in business because people will accept orders more easily from someone taller." So we expanded the club to include people who are small of stature.

I've also had transgender people joining—men who used to be women. They write that they'd be very happy to have the penis of the smallest guy in the club. It would be big in comparison to what they've got. So it just shows you there's always someone in a situation worse than yours.

PENIS SIZE IN ANCIENT GREECE AND ROME

There was one time and place we know of in human history when a small, dainty penis was considered to be the ideal. I'm speaking of Classical Athens. You can see it in their statues and vase paintings of nude men—the muscled torsos, the strong legs, the dear little cocks resting on sweet, modest balls. According to Eva C. Keuls in *The Reign of the Phallus*, a work of feminist scholarship, Athenians thought big sex organs were "coarse and ugly." But even they had their share of big-dick fantasies. Among their comic and erotic vase paintings are a horse and a bird with long, thick penises for heads, and a wide variety of satyrs whose large erections precede them.

21

Other pre-Christian cultures glorified big dicks, imagining huge ones for their fertility gods. One of the most compelling erotic images from the Roman Empire is a fresco of the fertility god, Priapus, discovered in the ruins of Pompeii. The handsome and well-built Priapus is dressed in a toga, standing at ease next to a basket of fruit. With one hand he lifts his skirt to give his very big, partly erect penis some air. In his other hand he holds a scale; the penis is resting on the scale, being weighed. It's a beautifully shaped cock, with a big head covered by a long, drooping foreskin, so you can't help staring at it and wondering what it can do—especially because its size is shocking. This image is so powerful, the guides at Pompeii tell the tourists, that little old ladies fall over backwards when they see it.

HOMOSEXUAL MEN

Homosexual men are connoisseurs of the penis. Not only do they have their own penises to think about; their lovers have penises as well. If size is important to heterosexual men, to homosexual men it's enormously important. To have a big dick, in the gay world, is automatically to be an object of desire. It's no accident that one of the most popular gay porn magazines is called *Inches*.

Those men who are most turned on by big dicks call themselves "size queens"—but penises have many qualities other than size, and there are men enough to admire each of these qualities. A gay friend explained some of the phallic fine distinctions to me: "There are some men who are not interested in any penis that is circumcised," he said. "Or, conversely, there are some who are only interested in penises that are circumcised. Some are absolutely completely rabid about large penises and will not even look at one that is medium or small. Some are only interested in small penises. I don't know why these fetishes exist, because I myself find all penises interesting—it's such an unusual organ and it has a life of its own.

"Some men are obsessed with curved penises. A curved penis can be fairly straight or it can be like a huge swoop. I think in general people like the upward swerve better than the downward swerve because it has a sort of exclamation point quality. I believe part of the interest in it is because it goes into the rectum in a curved way.

"And veined penises are very important, too. Veined penises are in the same category as muscles with veins. If you have veins it's a sinewy sort of thing—it's supposedly very masculine. Some men are only interested in a certain kind of a head of a penis, or a certain kind of uncircumcised penis. And the different kinds of heads . . . the most prized seeming to be a mushroom head as they call it, which is a head that's proportionally larger than the rest of the penis.

"I'd love to know how they discovered their obsessions. And how they meet people."

HETEROSEXUAL MEN

Unlike gay men, heterosexual men are not usually judged by their partners for penis size. On the whole women don't care that much about the size of a man's penis, as long as it fits reasonably well and he knows how to use it. Some women are size queens; most women appreciate a good-size dick if they happen to find themselves in bed with one—but they don't choose their men for the size of their dicks.

THE NATURE OF PENISES

You would think under the circumstances that heterosexual men would be relaxed about penis size, but this is
not the case. I'm not saying all men think about it all the
time, but I am saying it crops up. Once I was having dinner with a man I loved at a popular and crowded restaurant, and I made the mistake of ordering baby quail. Two
or three of these babies arrived on the plate, each about
the size and shape of a chicken egg. As I was about to start
cutting up the first one, my lover stopped me.

"Put the whole thing in your mouth," he said.

"What?" I said.

"Put the whole thing in your mouth."

"I don't think it will fit," I said.

He nudged me with his elbow. "If it doesn't fit," he
said, "everyone will think my cock isn't big enough."

There was no point trying to explain to him the difference between eating a baby quail and taking a man's
cock in your mouth; that the baby quail contains many
tiny bones and that once you've got it in your mouth you
need to chew it. He'd had a few drinks and was off in his
own mental jungle.

When it comes to gauging their erections, adult heterosexual men would have little to compare themselves
with if it weren't for pornography. Before the advent of pornographic films there were descriptions in porn novels of
men with huge members performing prodigious sexual
feats. Now a man can rent full-color vivid videos, and he
can see these heroes for himself. In the same way that fashion magazines set the standards for female beauty, X-rated
videos show men what the possibilities are in the realm of
genital appearance. And just as women starve themselves
to be thin, and get nose jobs and face-lifts, men are now
encouraged, by ads in newspapers and magazines and on
the Internet, to get themselves bigger dicks.

Porn stars, of course, are selected for size, staying power and ability to have erections on demand. You can see them fucking their way with aplomb through film after film, wielding their tools like hoses. Porn stars never get nervous on camera about their erections, they never hurry, they don't break stride. When they have orgasms their semen spurts out of them like milk from an udder. Their penises are mighty rods of flesh that gleam in the lights (and they're photographed from below to make them seem even bigger than they are). Female porn stars can't get enough of them. "Put that big fat cock inside my tight wet pussy," they say. "Ooh, baby, I'm so hot for your fat hard dick."

DO BIG DICKS
HAVE MORE FUN?

I interviewed a man in New York who's known to have a big penis, and asked him about his sex life.

A: The best thing I can say about having a big cock is you don't have to work so hard. It's a major contributor to laziness. You can just lie back there, whereas people with a certain complex in that area can become incredibly good technicians at cunnilingus and things like that.

Q: *When did you first become aware that you had a gift?*

A: Very young. I remember we wore short trousers at school. There was someone at a nearby school who was famous for his size. He wasn't allowed to wear short trousers. I was allowed to wear short trousers—I was nowhere near that length. But I got a hard-on in chapel when I was something under eleven. It was one of the first ones I'd ever got, and it was very noticeable. I was both embarrassed and rather delighted. You know, there's a definite downside, which is that when you're quite young, when you're first becoming sexually active, it's often very hard to fuck someone. The girls are not exactly virgins, but they're not relaxed. I've had a great many failures, when I was young and all through my life, with younger people.

Q: Do you need special-size condoms?

A: Size large. It seems to me that large size has suddenly started becoming available. In the old days when it was difficult to get the big ones I'd frequently break them, and the consequence could be pregnancy.

Q: Do big penises run in your family?

A: I have no idea. We didn't talk about that kind of thing.

Q: What are its dimensions?

A: I don't think it's ten inches or anything like that.

Q: Five to seven is normal.

A: Well, it's longer than that. But so what? I've known some really notorious womanizers, some of whose careers have been deformed by the extent of their obsessions. I don't know how big their cocks are and I'm not really interested, but I'm sure it's got nothing much to do with their obsession. I don't think they're abnormally big or small.

Q: But guys who are normal size want to know, does a guy with a big one have a better sex life than they do.

A: Just the other day I was at a party and a couple of women came up, screaming all over the place about my size, only one of whom had any right to the conversation, and this happens about once every three months, it's probably that often.

Q: Do you think women like you because of it?

A: Some people are more into the physical aspect of sex than others, some women and some men are totally dominated by that, and for such people it makes a difference. Have I in my life had women friends who loved me only for that? Probably yes.

Q: *Ever feel like a sex object?*

A: Men who complain about that are lying through their teeth.

WOMEN TALK ABOUT PENIS SIZE

"To me, penis size isn't anywhere near as important as the size of the brain."

"Size does matter. It's been ingrained that bigger is better, and a large man seems powerful in a really primal way. I've had normal-size men, and making love with them felt nice, it just wasn't wholeheartedly satisfying. My best lover to date was about eight and a half inches. Nine is probably my cutoff. I like them to be big around, also. There's something about proportion that's important. I'm a big, broad woman. I can't date short men, either. It all comes back to power. There's this minor bit of pain that's a powerful element with a bigger man. The sensation is deeper and there's less work involved. Sex can be extremely pleasurable without a lot of movement. That space is filled."

"When I was eighteen I was pretty promiscuous, and I hooked up with this punk-rock guy and I was so into him, and the rumor had it he had this huge cock, and it was pierced and all this good shit, and I was all psyched. I got with him, and it hurt. Let me tell you,

27

it was so big that I was like, Oh, no. It was so big it was a big problem. I thought, Damn. I was so excited, for this?"

"When you're in the heat of first love you're living in illusion, and his dick could be a pencil, it doesn't matter, because you supply all the rest. Then as you go on, if it *is* a pencil it matters, it really does."

"Men are so worried about length, but width is much more important. You can really feel a wide one."

"It doesn't have to be the biggest dick in the world. But if it's too small it kind of gets lost. Once you hit average, size doesn't matter from there on up. It depends on how good a lover they are."

"Just for fun I called up some escort services, to find out what they were offering and how much they charged. They said all their escorts had very big penises. 'How big?' I said. They said they were at least ten inches. I said, 'Ten inches, what is that? A murder weapon?'"

PENIS ENLARGEMENT SURGERY

Surgery on the penis is not a new idea. Men have been circumcising and castrating each other for centuries. A seventeenth-century Chinese novel mentioned in G. L. Simons's *The Phallic Mystique* has a scene in which a doctor who advertises penis enlargement explains his method. The doctor does it by adding slices of erect dog penis. He harvests the dog penis when it's inside a bitch and the dog is about to ejaculate, he says. He slices the dog penis off at the root, cuts it into quarters, inserts the quarters while still warm into incisions in the patient's penis, rubs the whole thing with ointment and wraps it in bandages. Three months later the new organ is ready to go to work, with erections twenty times the size of a normal man's.

In reality you can't augment a penis by slicing it open and adding something else, without also making the owner impotent. Modern penis enlargement surgery, which offers much more modest increases, was developed out of ex-perimental work done by pediatric urologists on infants with congenital defects. The two procedures, one to lengthen the penis, the other to add girth, were introduced to the general public in 1991. In mid-1997 one surgeon estimated that at least fifteen thousand in the U.S. had al-ready had their penises surgically enlarged. Among these men was the comic Flip Wilson, who claimed his penis needed enlargement because he'd worn it down with over-use. In August of 1997 Wilson gave the surgery its first celebrity endorsement when he pulled it out and showed it off to the people in the control booth on Howard Stern's radio show.

Dr. Jed Kaminetsky, a urologist who was the first to perform the surgery in New York City, and who has since stopped doing it, described the odd nature of the practice to me.

"Most of the people who came to me for this surgery had average-size penises. I measured all of them, flaccid and erect, before the surgery, and I photographed them. I had a whole cabinet of photographs. We had to induce an erection so we could measure it. I stocked up on gay porn because over fifty percent of the men who came in were gay. And I had straight porn for the other men. It's much easier for a woman to go buy gay porn than it is for a straight man. I sent my wife.

"A whole series of very macho guys came to see me—Rocky, and Bruno, macho Italian guys. I saw a lot of Asians who wanted the surgery. It just runs the gamut.

"There was one guy who came to me, and his penis looked like a beer can. I don't think he was using it to have sex with anyone. He had already had three or four penile enlargements. He kept having it revised and putting more girth on it. His penis was almost as wide as it was long. It was over six inches around in its flaccid state. He asked me to do more and I had to say no.

"That was one reason I stopped doing the surgery—the patients had too much emotional baggage. Also the results aren't great. The surgery isn't perfected yet, and in the end I didn't feel comfortable doing it or recommending it be done."

Because penis enlargement surgery is not perfected, both the American Urological Association and the American Society of Plastic and Reconstructive Surgeons refuse to endorse it. Medical schools don't teach it and textbooks don't describe it. But there are at least thirty doctors, worldwide, who perform the surgery on an outpatient basis—at a cost of nearly $6,000 if lengthening and widening are done at the same time, and with varying degrees of success.

The standard penis lengthening procedure entails cutting the suspensory ligament that holds the penis at a particular angle to the pubic bone. Freed of this ligament, the logic goes, the penis can dangle farther down out of the body. Surgeons promise one to two and a half inches of increased length, and then prescribe the wearing of weights a few hours every day for several months, to keep the extra piece of penis from retreating back inside.

Extra girth—up to 50 percent more, some surgeons say—can be added in one of two ways. A few years ago surgeons favored liposuction. They would suction fat out of the patient's abdomen and insert it into the penis. This is the same method that is used to add pout to women's lips, and it was invented by the same man who invented lip liposuction. It has the same drawback, too—eventually some of the fat gets reabsorbed, and the procedure must be repeated.

A newer method is the dermal fat graft: The surgeon removes a strip of dermis, or skin layer, from the buttocks or thigh, and sews it into the penis. This is more permanent, but it is also a more complicated operation. Still, it's now the only widening procedure some surgeons will do. Too often when liposuctioned fat is injected into the penis it distributes itself unevenly, forming lumps. Imagine a man who used to worry that his penis was too thin. He has the surgery and now it's fatter, but lumpy. Not only is he embarrassed to have sex, he's so angry he initiates a malpractice suit. In one case I read about the doctor seemed indignant that he was being sued. Nothing was wrong, he said. The patient just needed to massage the lumps vigorously enough, and eventually everything would even out.

Lumpy penis is only one of the surgery's possible side effects. Sometimes the lengthening procedure actually ends up shortening the penis, and usually it decreases the angle of the erection. Either surgery can cause scarring, numbness, blood vessel damage and impotence. It's somewhat safer to have your penis lengthened, wait a few months and then have it widened. But proceeding that way is more expensive—lengthening alone costs close to $4,000 and widening can be as much as $5,000.

Of course, many men have had the surgery without complications, and some of them have been interviewed for magazine articles in which they say they're much happier now. Most likely they're men who had really small penises to start with, for whom an extra inch would be a big percentage gain. As for the rest, according to Dr. Kaminetsky, "You can add length, but not that much erect length, so basically it makes guys look better in the shower. Nobody I operated on was really unhappy afterward. But I don't think it changed anybody's life, I'll tell you that."

PUMPING IT UP

Any man who reads men's magazines has seen ads for penis enlargement vacuum pumps, in the back of the book near the hair transplant ads. The first penis pumps were patented around 1914; they were invented to help men get and maintain erections, and even after the advent of Viagra, modern versions are still sometimes used for that purpose. Dr. Kaminetsky, many of whose patients have erection problems, showed me a vacuum pump when I visited his office. It was a clear plastic cylinder, longer and wider than any ordinary penis, open at one end and sealed at the other. A tube coming out of the sealed end was attached to a suction pump. Dr. Kaminetsky told me to put my palm over the open end of the cylinder he was holding. He pumped air out of the cylinder, and I could feel the strong pull on my palm. A penis, inserted into the tube, would be pulled in the same way: As air is pumped out the penis expands to fill the space.

A pump is a cumbersome treatment for impotence. The couple must wait until the man pumps up and removes himself from the tube before their lovemaking can proceed, and then his erection will be big and heavy rather than stiff, "like a cold sausage," as Dr. Kaminetsky put it.

But a man alone with his pump can get a thrill just from watching his organ grow.

Men who pump can devote hours to the equipment, discuss the fine points with fellow pumpers, tune in to other people's experiences at various web sites on the Internet, look at pictures of other people's pumping results. And all the while the equipment, shaped somewhat like a penis, is meant to enhance *their* equipment, the penis itself.

This pumping is no simple operation. First of all there's the question of what kind of pump to buy: cheap or expensive, manual or electric. And then, when you use it, should the tube be filled with hot water (not if it's electric it shouldn't)? And what kind of lubricant should you use? (One man wrote to his fellows at a pumping web site, "I use olive oil for lube. It's all natural, inexpensive, great for your skin and washes off the tubes with a drop of detergent.") And how long and at what pressure should you pump? And after you're pumped up should you keep it on while you watch TV (lots of pumpers do)? And should you ejaculate into it (you'll have to clean it)? And how long should your penis stay big after it's thoroughly pumped (several hours, some say)? And is it a good idea to tell your wife about your practice? And, most important, will pumping affect your erections? These and other questions are debated at length on the Internet.

Many pumpers trim their pubic hair before pumping —to get a good seal, some say, and also to make their penises look bigger. They use different-size cylinders: a longer, thinner one to expand length, and a shorter, wider one to expand width. Some men pump their balls. Some use a "cock cushion," a thick silicone ring placed around the base of the penis to restrict circulation and keep it from deflating totally between meetings with the vacuum tube. A man who devotes several hours a day to pumping his penis may be able to keep it in a perpetually pumped-up state. On the other hand, if he pumps too much he could lose his ability to have natural erections.

In spite of what pumpers like to believe, there is no scientific evidence that pumping permanently enlarges the penis. But in the end this detail may be unimportant. No one becomes a pumper who doesn't enjoy it. Though it is done with a goal in mind and might be thought of as exercise, pumping is also, it must be said, a form of sexual activity. That's why one manufacturer advertises "The Electric Deep Throat Developer System," with fifty "throbbing, root-milking pulses per minute. . . . Develop your cock to stud-like proportions and get the ultimate suck job at the same time."

WEIGHING IT DOWN

I was at a party the first time I heard about penis weights. A few of us were sitting around a coffee table, balancing plates of food on our knees, and John said he had a friend who wore weights on his penis to make it bigger. Sometimes this friend wore his weights to the office. He worked, John said, as a bond trader on Wall Street.

"Wall Street—no wonder," Michael said. "They call the hotshot traders there Big Swinging Dicks."

It was hard to imagine how a man could go to the office with a weight on his penis. Eventually someone would notice it under his pants. Or somebody would bump into him and feel it—a three-pound metal ball hooked by a rope to the corona just above the head of his penis, dangling halfway down to his knees.

But maybe this man was actually wearing a Yank Super Stretcher. This is made of elastic and is advertised as something you can keep on discreetly all day long. An elastic band fits around the corona and is attached by means of elastic to another band around the thigh so that it exerts a constant pull.

The Yank, which costs only $18.50, is the most elementary of stretchers. Upscale from the Yank are several makes with a ring that fits around the base of the penis, another ring that fits over the head, and rods of adjustable length running between the two rings to keep the penis in a state of constant anxiety. Stretchers can cost as much as $900.

Men who use weights have probably been encouraged by stories brought back from India and Africa. The Indian sadhus, for example, are said to put some of their boys on a regimen of penis weight training from the age of six. By the time these boys reach manhood their penises are extraordinarily long—and correspondingly thin. The chosen adult sadhus wear their penises knotted up inside cloth baskets. They believe a lengthened penis brings a man closer to god. When it comes to sexual intercourse, they're useless.

MILKING IT

There are also old-fashioned manual methods of penis enlargement, for those who would rather masturbate. The most intriguing of these is "jelq," practiced by the Sudanese Arabs, who are supposedly well hung as a consequence. When a boy is eight, the story goes, his father passes on to him the secrets of jelq, showing him how to take his penis between thumb and forefinger and, using medium-firm pressure and long strokes, to milk it from base to tip, hand over hand. The boy learns to stop the massage when he comes close to ejaculation, wait for the feeling to subside, then start again; he practices for a half hour a day, approaching ejaculation six or seven times. If the family has money the boy may be sent to a "mehbil," or athletic club, where an attendant, after massaging him with oil, will do the jelq for him.

Jelq is most effective when initiated during boyhood, according to Gary Griffin, MBA, the American Pied Piper for penis enlargement, but grown men can benefit from the practice, if they're willing to devote themselves to it for a year or more. Griffin, author of twelve books about the penis, describes jelq, and many other paths to enlargement, in *Penis Enlargement Methods—Fact & Phallusy*. In his opinion the real frontier in penis enlargement may be hypnosis and autosuggestion. When this method is perfected, if all goes well, a man may be able to imagine himself with the dick of his dreams so fervently and consistently that eventually his body will respond by growing it.

TWO COMPARATIVE STUDIES OF PENISES

A NUDE BEACH

One of my informants took me to a low-key nudist beach in Sandy Hook, New Jersey. Among the beachgoers were families, heterosexual couples, gay couples. A lot of promenading went on, as it does on any beach, and as on any beach a majority of the promenaders were men. There they were, strolling and talking, as their dicks bobbed along on their balls or dangled meekly between their legs. Some looked like flower buds, some looked like pencils, some looked like faucets, some looked like mushrooms, some looked like sausages—and they all looked like each other. Flaccid and out in the open they seemed terribly vulnerable.

After a trip to a nudist beach you can see men in business clothes striding down city sidewalks and imagine them inside their suits as if they were vulnerable nudists.

GAY PINUP MAGAZINES

My first time shopping at a magazine store in the section for gay porn and pinup magazines I riffled through the available merchandise—*Jock, Mandate, Bunkhouse, Stallion, Bear* (for people who like hairy, portly, manly men), *Foreskin Quarterly* and so on. Fighting off my dread of being thought sexually weird, I stepped up to the counter and bought *Playgirl* and *Inches*. *Playgirl* was supposed to be for women. As for *Inches,* I liked its name. I bought it even though it had a picture on the cover of a man in bright white Jockey shorts. Much as I love men, I do not understand the appeal of Jockey shorts. They remind me of my older brother—whom I love, but to whom I have never been sexually attracted—who used to wear them around the house when I thought he should be dressed. Sometimes they had mysterious stains on them.

When I got these magazines home I left them alone for a while. Enrique came over and I showed them to him. He said he couldn't look. Then later I found him slowly turning the pages of one of them, holding it at arm's length, shaking his head. "Ai, caramba, these are major pieces of meat," he said. I dipped into them. A friend loaned me some back issues of *Inches* and of a more specialized offshoot publication, *Black Inches*. They just brought out the prude in me.

Sheltered as I was, I'd never seen such a forest of dicks before. Fear came up; fear and disinclination. Most women

37

aren't all that turned on by anonymous body parts—we respond better if there's a nice, romantic story. But here, you open a gay pinup magazine, and a naked guy you've never seen before is ogling you. He's dumb as milk, he has this awful come-on look and he's pressing his pelvis forward, presenting to you for your delectation his big, hard-as-a-ramrod cock. The covers of my magazines advertised the riches inside: "Super Top Blade Thompson's Uncut Crotch Muscle," "Rico's 10–Inch Jawbreaker" and much, much more. These were phenomena I did and did not want to know about. I sat down and looked at them, until my resistance disappeared.

I saw a man with a stockbroker's haircut and pale skin, lightly tanned all over, who had a rosy pink erection that stood straight out, curving downward ever so slightly, like a dowsing rod. A man with swarthier skin had a glistening prick of a uniform coral color. An African-American man, muscled and bronze-colored, had a thick, uncircumcised dick as dark as bittersweet chocolate. One man, called "Black Thunder," was brown all over, with a very long, wide penis that curved in the middle and had a beautiful pink head, the same color as his belly button. When I paid attention to them I began to feel a kind of affection for these penises, and even a bit of lust.

The best photographs were the ones where the men were not looking at the camera, but at their penises; their expressions were tender and amused. In one series of pictures the man seemed almost to be dancing with his penis—which was fat, veined and uncircumcised. Dancing, or playing, or letting it have its way, he was seeing what it might do when it was on its own, as if it were his pet, or his baby brother.

Those pictures are often in my mind. It seems so right when a man's penis brings out his good nature. When that happens, size is totally beside the point.

PART

TWO

PENIS

CULTURE

*O*ne of the first things I wanted to know about penises—after looking into the size issue, which weighs so heavily upon our minds and culture—was whether they had always been taboo. The answer turned out to be, not at all. Some cultures, ancient and modern, can't get enough of penises—they worship them, sculpt them, wear them as pendants. Others, like our present Judeo-Christian culture, consider it best for all concerned to keep them hidden. Few if any have been nonchalant about penises, for obvious reasons.

Right now we seem to be moving toward an easy familiarity with the subject. To help you adjust your sights, this section brings you visible penises—erect if possible—from various times and places, in religion, the arts, fashion and popular culture.

CHAPTER
THREE

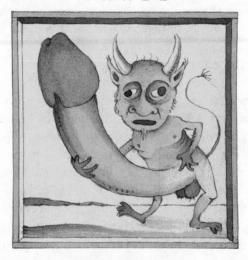

PENIS
WORSHIP

Men have always been proud of their penises, but before Christianity they used to be more open about it. From the Neolithic period, when men discovered their role in conception, until Christianity spread through Europe, almost every culture had gods with visible penises. Not only visible, but huge.

The Greeks liked penises so much they had a number of penis gods—Priapus was one, Dionysus was another, Hermes another—in fact Hermes is a word for penis in Greek. Bacchus—also known as Liber—was the native Roman penis god. Osiris was the Egyptian penis god. Shiva was the Indian penis god, and there is still a lingam chapel devoted to Shiva in every Hindu temple. In ancient places as various and widespread as India, Japan, Greece, Rome and Britain, there were festivals every year in honor of the penis gods. Huge dummy penises were carried through the streets, people wore penis masks and the feasts usually ended in orgies. Women were often major participants. During the festivals housewives got to wear fake phalluses and behave like men. Then they went back to their circumscribed lives.

When the penis gods reigned, phallic monuments littered the landscape. Egyptians erected obelisks, those lofty squared-off phalluses with pyramid tips. Some survive—among them a Cleopatra's Needle relocated to New York's Central Park and another to London's Embankment. (The Washington Monument, more than forty stories high, is the nineteenth-century American version.) In Dorset, England, the Cerne Abbas giant, thought to date from the second century A.D., is clearly visible today. An enormous drawing cut in chalk on to a green hill, the giant wields a gigantic club and sports an erection that stretches from balls to belly button. The entire figure covers so much ground that a couple of humans can easily have intercourse within the bounds of the phallus. Over the centuries many have done so, hoping for fertility and good luck. On the Greek Island of Delos the remains of the Avenue of Priapus can still be seen—huge stone phalluses perched atop carved stone pillars like cannons aiming gism at the stars.

In societies that practiced phallic worship, phalluses often adorned everyday objects. They were common in the vase paintings of Classical Greece, which regularly took sex play as their subject—between mortals, and among mortals, satyrs and gods. In the excavated ruins of Pompeii the phallus was a leitmotif. There were bronze ornaments in the shape of phalluses with bells hanging from them; gaily winged phalluses with phallic legs and tails; terracotta bowls with phalluses jutting from them; lamps made of faunlike figures weighed down by huge dick wicks. The ancient Peruvian Mochica culture made a specialty of pitchers with phalluses for spouts. These objects, in which the penis is either disembodied or disproportionately huge, give it an unseemly gravity. If you lived among these objects as a woman you would probably experience penises in some ways more the way men do; they wouldn't seem alien to you, but on the other hand you'd be forced to think about them all the time.

Penises, apparently so magical, were widely thought to ward off the evil eye. Small sculptures of phalluses were found on the exterior walls of houses in Pompeii (and can be seen today on the walls of houses in Sikkim). In ancient Rome a victorious general would suspend a huge phallus on his chariot, to insure that success would not destroy his luck. Ancient Romans wore phallic amulets around their necks, or on a bracelet, to protect themselves. Some of these were penis-shaped, others were in the shape of a fist with the middle finger extended, or a fist with the thumb protruding between the second and ring fingers. Those hand symbols are still worn for good luck, though some wearers may not know what they really symbolize. The Latin word for these magical representations of the penis is *fascinum*—the origin of the English word "fascinate."

Vulvas were also used as good-luck symbols in some cultures. It's easy for me to imagine that men are reminded of their destiny and their importance when they see a phallus being worshiped. Because that's the way I felt when I saw drawings of the Shelah-na-Gig, the Medieval Irish vulva symbol. To my surprise I was proud that vulvas were esteemed for their life-enhancing properties, and were sculpted on the outsides of Irish churches.

Vulvas were not at all as widely revered as penises, and this is probably because men were in charge. It would be wrong to say that men were in charge *because* they had penises—the reasons are much more complicated, and strength and capacity for violence are more to the point. But erect penises were a symbol of the authority of men, reminding everyone that a man with an erection was a person full of fervor and determination; a person who might be dangerous.

PHALLIC TALES

Though female gods often represented the earth, from the Neolithic period onward the gods responsible for creation were always male. Sometimes the penis of a god or ruler figured in his mythology. Penises of men and statues also might have ritual or magical properties.

MYTHS AND LEGENDS

In Greek mythology it was said that Chronos, son of the Titan Uranus, castrated his father and threw his penis into the sea. Although this was not a happy event for Uranus, it was good for humanity. Aphrodite, Goddess of Love, rose from the sea where Uranus's penis had fertilized the waters.

The Egyptian hero Osiris was slain in battle and cut into pieces by his enemy, Typhon. Typhon's followers took the pieces, with Typhon himself keeping the phallus. Then Isis, wife of Osiris, gained control of the government and rounded up the pieces of her husband. Only the penis could not be found—Typhon had apparently fled with it, and may have thrown it in the sea. In honor of Osiris, Isis ordered that the phallus be worshiped with solemnities and mysteries. Osiris's misfortune became the origin of phallus worship among the Egyptians.

The Chinese emperor Chou-hsin was said to be a sexual prodigy. His penis was supposedly so big and strong he could walk around a room with a naked woman perched on his erection. He lived by the precept of the Yellow Emperor, copulating with ten women every night without ejaculating (or "losing the Vital Essence," as it was called). Eventually he became impotent—at which point he beheaded the medical advisor who had counseled him to conduct himself in such a manner.

According to Plutarch, Rome was founded by the offspring of a disembodied phallus and a servant girl. The phallus appeared one day in the fireplace of the King of Albani. The king ordered his daughter to copulate with the phallus, but the princess sent her maidservant instead. The maidservant did as she was told, and the phallus impregnated her. Her two sons, Romulus and Remus, whom she abandoned in the forest to be fed by wolves, became the fathers of Rome.

KARNAK

The Egyptian god of creation was Amun, to whom the Temple at Karnak is dedicated. Built during the XVIII dynasty, which lasted from 1501 to 1342 B.C., and excavated in the nineteenth century by Napoleon's armies, the temple is still the largest columned building in the world, with two 330-ton obelisks out front, enormous statues, long corridors, rooms within rooms. It's also one of the world's major tourist attractions.

Ancient Egyptians believed Amun created the world each day out of watery chaos by masturbating and swallowing his own semen, then spitting it out. It's not entirely clear whether Amun used his hand for this task or performed autofellatio. There are many bas-reliefs on the temple walls of figures with big erect penises; in at least one of these a figure lying flat on his back with his legs folded over toward his head is about to take his own very long phallus into his mouth. But Amun's hand was certainly important.

Apparently each day, in the innermost temple, Amun's shrine, the original act of creation would be ritually reenacted. Nobody knows exactly what this means, but archaeologists are willing to imagine. Originally they thought a statue of the god standing up was used in the rituals, but now they think the ritual statue was the one where the god is sitting; he has a flail in his right hand and in his left he grips his big, erect dick. The walls are as high as men can see. This is obviously a holy place, but what does "holy" mean here?

When the priests performed their ceremonies, their whole bodies were first shaven, then bathed. They oiled and clothed the god. They brought him incense and dancing girls, anything to stimulate him to reenact creation one more time. Other than that we don't know what they did, exactly. It may have been something symbolic, but we'd all like to think it was something sexual. The high priestess probably had something to do with it, in her role as the wife of the god. The wife of the god had another title: God's Hand.

THE HERMS

Athens in fifth century B.C. was a capital of phallic power, and one manifestation of the city's rampant phallicism was its high concentration of herms. Named for the god Hermes, herms were vertical stone slabs with sculptures of the bearded head of Hermes on top and protruding sculpted erections at penis level. The herms stood in front of private houses and at street corners; they marked boundaries between properties; they massed together in the marketplace, jutting out at each other and every pass-erby. Their presence was thought to protect the populace from evil, and individuals routinely touched the erections for good luck. Then one night in 415 B.C., as the men of Athens were preparing to sail to Sicily for a new foray against the Spartans in the continuing Peloponnesian War, someone chopped the dicks off all the herms. Bad luck ensued; Athens lost to Sparta. The herm-choppers were never found, and although this happened 2,500 years ago, for some strange reason it's still being discussed. In *The Reign of the Phallus,* Eva Keuls builds an elaborate case to show that it must have been the respectable women, con-fined to the women's quarters of the house, who castrated the herms in the dead of night, to make the point that phallicism had gone too far.

SWEARING

Nowadays Western people swear on the Bible, but before there were Bibles, men used to swear on their penises, or on the penises of the men they were swearing to. In the Bible when men swear, the translators euphe-mistically refer to the penis as a thigh. Here are two ex-amples from Genesis: Abraham asking his servant to swear to him: "'Put your hand under my thigh, and I will make you swear by the Lord, the God of heaven and of earth,'" (Gen. 24: 2–3). And Jacob on his deathbed: "He called his son Joseph and said to him, 'If now I have found favor in your sight, put your hand under my thigh, and promise to deal loyally and truly with me,'" (Gen. 47: 29).

It may be that "thigh" really means testicles, or penis and testicles. In any case the word "testify" comes from this practice.

PENIS CULTURE

DEFLOWERING VIRGINS

Christianity could banish all the penis gods, but it couldn't stamp out penis magic. In Europe throughout the Middle Ages people wore phallic amulets, drew phalluses on their churches and sought the protection of certain Christian saints who had inherited the phallic powers of the former gods—for example, St. Foutin, who was popular in the South of France, Provence, Languedoc and the Lyonnais. A medieval statue of St. Foutin was likely to be furnished with a large, erect wooden phallus. Barren women would scrape this phallus, steep the scrapings in water and drink the mixture in the hope it would make them fertile, or give it to their husbands to drink to improve their potency. Statues of other saints with prominent phalluses—Gilles, Arnaud, Guignole—were also appealed to with a scraping knife. The saintly penises, worn down by constant attention, would from time to time experience miraculous renewals. "The phallus consisted of a long staff of wood passed through a hole in the middle of the body," says Thomas Wright in his 1866 classic, *The Worship of the Generative Powers*, "and as the phallic end in front became shortened, a blow of a mallet from behind thrust it forward, so that it was restored to its original length." The practice of asking phallic statues of saints for help with fertility continued in some places well into the eighteenth century.

In another related practice in Medieval Europe certain statues of phallic saints were used during wedding ceremonies to deflower the brides. This custom originated in ancient times when a statue of Priapus would do the deed. The purpose in both cases was to insure good fortune and fertility. In *The Worship of the Generative Powers*, Wright says he believes that intercourse with statues of saints is what inspired women in the use of artificial phalluses for sexual gratification, "a vice which is understood to prevail especially in nunneries."

Using statues to deflower virgins was still common practice in the nineteenth century in India, Japan and the Pacific Islands. "Even today," Alain Danielou wrote in 1993 in *The Phallus,* "the young girls of Nepal have their hymens broken by means of a phallus-shaped fruit in a rite that grants to the god a sort of 'droit du seigneur.'"

THE DEVIL'S DICK

Witches' Sabbaths of the Middle Ages, which were described as large-scale orgies, probably descended from the phallic cults. Celebrants worshiped a horned god who, at least in the minds of the Inquisitors who brought the witches to trial, represented the devil. Like Priapus, the devil was often said to have a huge penis, and celebrants were said to have sex with him. His semen, they reported, was ice-cold. If nothing else the broomstick was a phallic symbol. Wright describes the way witches proceeded: "They took an ointment given to them by the devil, with which they anointed a wooden rod, at the same time rubbing the palms of their hands with it, and then, placing the rod between their legs, they were suddenly carried through the air to the place of assembly."

Beguiled by the devil's dick, witches were thought to have power over the penises of ordinary men. During the Inquisition, people who were accused of witchcraft were often said to have made men impotent, or even caused their penises to disappear. (The spell a witch was said to cast to disappear a penis was called a "glamour"—the origin of our word for magical appeal.) The following is from a translation of *Malleus Maleficarum,* the fifteenth-century book on witchcraft that was a basic text of the Inquisition: "For a certain man tells that, when he had lost his member, he approached a known witch to ask her to restore it to him. She told the afflicted man to climb a certain tree, and that he might take which he liked out of a nest in which there were several members. And when he tried to take a big one, the witch said: 'You must not take that one'; adding, 'because it belonged to a parish priest.'"

IDEAS ABOUT PROCREATION

So convinced was everyone of the godlike nature of the penis and its products, so marvelous an instrument did it seem to be, that from 9000 B.C. until the eighteenth century most people believed that babies came from semen alone. Men planted the seed; women were simply the earth in which it grew. Semen contained everything necessary to make a man. People believed this even though children often looked like their mothers.

With the invention of the microscope in the seventeenth century scientists discovered that semen teemed with tiny creatures, which we call sperm and they called animalcules or homunculi, because they looked like minuscule people. A human, then, was a homunculus that got planted and grew. During the eighteenth century, botanists proved that in the case of plants both parents were responsible for the characteristics of the offspring. It wasn't until 1854 that the fusion of frog sperm and egg was seen under a microscope and the basic facts of animal reproduction became absolutely clear. The suffragist movement began at about the same time. I'm not suggesting cause and effect—only that some discoveries can't be made until the climate is right for their acceptance.

CONTEMPORARY PENIS WORSHIP

Today, if you want to experience organized phallic worship you have to go to Japan, or find a Hindu temple. For the personal kind, there are still men around—Enrique met one recently—who say things like, "I expect women to worship at the altar of my cock." But that's another story.

JAPANESE PHALLUS FESTIVALS

Shinto, the original Japanese religion, was a nature religion, and phallic worship was worship of the life force. Apparently, Japan is full of naturally occurring, penis-shaped stones, and these are thought to have magical, protective powers. There are shrines to phallic stones all over the country. In 1953 there were 420 phallic stones extant in Nagano Prefecture and 14 in Tokyo alone.

Phallicism is mostly a rural religion now—in practice, a farmer and his wife might make love in a field while the seed is being sown to insure a good crop; or a couple might spend a night with the silkworms to encourage them to spin.

There are also various local fertility festivals with phallic elements. As recently as 1953, at a festival in Chiba, right near Tokyo, a wooden phallus would have ritual sex with a straw vagina, after which they would be anointed with milky rice beer. In Tohoku a basketware phallus covered in red papier-mâché was paraded through the streets once a year to purify the air. In Hakata they would build a phallus as big as a house, set it on fire and throw it into the sea.

Each year during a phallus festival at the 1,500-year-old Tagata Shrine, a new seven-foot penis carved from a

51

Japanese cypress, and weighing some seven hundred pounds, is carried by twelve men from the Kumano Shrine, a mile up the road, to the Tagata Shrine. The phallus is so heavy that several teams of twelve are needed. After appropriate ceremonies the phallus of the year is placed in a room with other attending phalluses, and last year's specimen can then be sold. This festival, meant to promote fertility and prosperity and protect against evil, is a tourist favorite.

In some towns there are festivals during which young men wear protective phalluses carved of daikon radishes on their belts. Many local festivals sell penis-shaped talismans, some of which—like a boat with a phallic mast—are used as children's toys.

In some cases just the sight of the penis can be enough to root out evil. A May festival in Kyoto was dedicated to an ugly goddess who tried to break up young lovers. In order to quiet the goddess, the young men of the district would carry her on a palanquin through the streets; they wore only short coats and no loincloths, so she could plainly see their penises. In a town called Bingo, if the rice pot bubbled too much on the stove, the man of the house would expose himself to the pot. The pot would calm down.

There are a number of local New Year's festivals during which young men hit young women with carved phalluses or phallic-shaped objects in order to wish them good luck.

THE HINDU LINGAM CEREMONY

In Hinduism—the major religion of India—the phallic god Shiva, who represents the creative principle and the origin of all things, is worshiped in the form of his lingam, or penis. Hindu sacred art is often erotic, and includes many representations of penises, some of them sculpted on the outsides of temples. Shiva lingams inside temples aren't penis-shaped exactly; most of them look more like wide, flat, oval stones, or like fat, squat candles. In lingam-conscious India, lingams are also found in nature; the most famous is an ice stalagmite ten feet high inside the Amarnatha Cave, a major pilgrimage site.

My own experience with a Shiva lingam was at a Hindu temple in Flushing, New York—and it was Enrique, who came with me, who got the most out of it. The temple was an airy place to stroll through, with chapels for various gods and goddesses, and niches for statuettes of gods and goddesses who didn't have chapels. Signs said "Please do not touch the Deity." It was early evening. We sat cross-legged on the floor along with some Indian women in saris and men in business clothes, in front of the lingam chapel. A small statue of a sitting bull, on a stand, also faced the chapel. When the ceremony began the chapel curtain was pulled to reveal a big, oval, reddish green lingam, set in a yoni, a vulva-shaped basin, so that the top two thirds of the lingam were visible.

(Apparently there's a bull facing the Shiva lingam in every temple in India, and the painter Rackstraw Downes told me a tale about this configuration that he heard from a guide in the ancient city of Hampi. Shiva, the story goes, was in the mood for sex one day. However, his lover, Parvati, was not receptive, and he was forced to resort to the bull in the field. Shiva promised the bull that after he screwed it, he would let it screw him. The bull agreed. Shiva took his pleasure with the bull, and ever since the bull has sat there, waiting for its turn.)

Two young priests officiated at the Flushing chapel. They were naked on top and wore white lengths of cloth, wrapped around the waist, like figures on an ancient frieze.

Their work consisted mainly of pouring libations over the lingam, and over the bull. Among the offerings were milk, honey, yogurt, clarified butter and cut-up bananas, apples and oranges. After each new substance offered, the lingam and the bull were washed down with water. A bell was rung between offerings; a flower was placed on the lingam where its forehead would be if it were a face. All the while the men in the congregation chanted in Sanskrit.

I enjoyed watching the ceremony, but didn't get much of a charge from it. Enrique, on the other hand, was thrilled. He said it was like the Catholic Church, only better. There was the same tang of incense in your nostrils, and the chant droning in your brain; there were bells and candles—but instead of worshiping the Father, the Son and the Holy Ghost, you could celebrate the generative principle and its connection to your own maleness. Just the sort of thing Christianity wiped out and replaced in the West, two thousand years ago.

THE GENERATIVE PRINCIPLE

Enrique said a man could look at the lingam as a kind of model. "Because to accomplish anything you must penetrate. You penetrate other people's consciousness, or you take a seed and push it into the ground, and that's the beginning of anything you do. So the generative principle permeates absolutely everything. And isn't it fun? You can see it in a banal, silly piece of flesh plumbing. Through that silly piece of flesh plumbing comes anybody who's walked this earth."

CHAPTER

FOUR

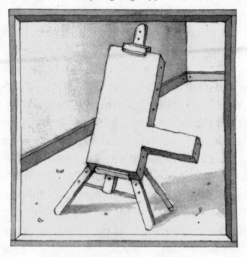

PENISES
IN ART

Before Christianity, Western art had its fair share of penises. Ordinary men were painted or sculpted with ordinary penises and gods were made with big, godlike erections. But in the respectable art of the Judeo-Christian West, which abounds in female nudes, erect penises have been conspicuously absent. Even flaccid penises aren't easy to find in the publicly accessible holdings of the grand Western museums.

At the Metropolitan Museum of Art in New York, for example, there is no armor for the penis in the armor collection; the armor has an arch and a space where the piece to protect the penis should be, but the piece is missing. There are one or two small and barely discernible penises on friezes in the Egyptian wing, though it's clear the ancient Egyptians were not shy about showing erections. There are no penises on the Greek vase paintings, and no adult penises in the European painting galleries, aside from two paintings of men with hard-to-make-out codpieces. There are some cherubs and Cupids whose baby dicks you can see, and a fair number of renditions of the baby Jesus' penis. Most modern people, though, when they look at paintings of the baby Jesus, don't think of his penis as a penis. (In the Renaissance, as Leo Steinberg demonstrates in an exhilarating monograph, *The Sexuality of Christ in Renaissance Art and in Modern Oblivion,* the motive was theological. Painting after painting shows the baby Jesus sitting on his mother's lap, his penis exposed, his mother pointing to it with pride. His penis is proof that he has "embodied himself in a human nature," becoming "mortal and sexual" for the sake of mankind.)

In the section of the museum devoted to tribal art there's only one exhibition with a bunch of realistically juicy dicks. These belong to some life-size figures made for the death ritual of the Asmat people of New Guinea. The figures are carved standing, one on the shoulders of another, and the carvings are placed outside the house of someone who dies. When a head-hunting expedition takes place, fresh heads are placed in the gaps in the sculpture. The standing figures have hefty, hanging-down penises.

The only other dicks are on nude Greek and Roman statues. Some of them are small and quiescent, with carved pubic hair and baby balls. The rest have been broken off.

When the Metropolitan Museum showed the larger-than-life-size male nudes of the English painter Lucian Freud, they put up a sign warning there would be nudity, even though none of the nudes had an erection. No such sign would be necessary for a show containing female nudes; female nudes are all over the museum.

Obviously, up until recent years most Western men have not wanted to represent penises, particularly erect penises, in their art; they also have not wanted to show the art of other cultures in which penises are prominent. One way of seeing this phenomenon is in terms of who does the looking and who is looked at. Traditionally women have been the objects and men have painted them or owned the paintings. Renoir's famous retort, when asked by a journalist how he could paint with his crippled hands, was "I paint with my prick." Like the sex act, in which the man is always said to possess the woman and never the other way around, such an arrangement can be seen as an expression of power. It's a different sort of expression from the exuberant erections of pagan times. We think of it as more civilized and therefore less threatening—but all it is, really, is more covert.

And the male position of powerful nondisclosure exacted a price; it made men afraid to show what they're really like—and men and women afraid to see them naked. In the art world of the late 1990s this position has come seriously unraveled.

FAMOUS ARTISTS DO EROTICA

Through the ages great artists as well as lesser ones have drawn and painted erections and sex acts of various kinds. But in the Judeo-Christian West these works were considered to be pornography. Many are privately owned, and most of the rest are held by museums in special collections. In recent years, with the relaxing of censorship, these works have also become widely available in anthologies of erotic art. Some of the artists whose work can be found in these anthologies include Leonardo da Vinci (a cross-section of a couple fucking); Parmigianino (I've seen an engraving of a Witches' Sabbath, where celebrants sit on a huge erect cock with the rump of a goat); Thomas Rowlandson (a series of bawdy etchings done around 1810, including one scene in Kensington Gardens of a bunch of phalluses with legs); Giulio Romano, who in Mantua decorated a room in the palazzo of Duke Federico II with a ceilingful of erotic frescoes; Aubrey Beardsley, George Grosz, Egon Schiele, Hans Bellmer, André Masson, Félicien Rops, Toulouse-Lautrec, Cocteau, Dali and Picasso. More often than not in this erotic work the penis is seen as either comical (the disembodied phalluses) or a cause of embarrassment and shame. (George Grosz and Egon Schiele both did self-portraits while masturbating. Schiele looks hollow-eyed and haunted; Grosz is shamefaced in the shadows, ejaculating while two women perform for him. The phalluses, the active elements in both portraits, are huge, throbbing and red.) Picasso often drew penises, erect and flaccid, and his work often dealt with sexual relationships. Because he was Picasso, and anything he made was assumed to be high art, his erotic works were shown in museums and sold in galleries. In 1997, when the Museum of Modern Art in New York had a large Schiele show, full of penises and vulvas, a lot of writers got to speculate in print about genitals as fit subjects for artists.

PENIS ART
IN THE 1990S

Even before "penis" the word began showing up in newspapers and on television in the mid-1990s, the image of the penis had started to appear in New York galleries. The photographs of Pierre Molinier, a French cross-dressing surrealist with a dildo obsession, came into vogue. Andres Serrano showed photographs of couples in which the men as well as the women were naked and aroused. There were so many group shows of erotic images, male and female, that critics began to say they were boring. Nevertheless, a great many people visited galleries to see them.

On the most basic level, an artwork with an erection in it dares the viewer to really look at this thing she's been taught not to think about. The act of viewing such an artwork expands the viewer's visual vocabulary and the ways in which he can think about male sexuality. Artists who work with penises, while using the image itself, are also playing with taboo and the idea of taboo, and with erotic charge and the idea of erotic charge.

For many people it's still jolting, or titillating, to find an erection in an art gallery, no matter what critics say. I asked one heterosexual man in the art business, who's in his forties, what he thought about all those dicks on gallery walls.

He said, "I think one of the last bastions of the male mysteries is the hard-on, and there's some sort of protection of that, we want it to remain a secret."

"You mean seeing an erection up on the wall is annoying?"

"I think it alerts one's senses," he said, "in a 'Maybe I'm about to beat the shit out of that guy' kind of way. There's a certain just animal sensation of 'What is he doing here?' It would be wrong to say one has no feeling about it. I do."

So if hiding erections is a power position, why are they coming out now? The answer must be that more than wanting power of the patriarchal kind, some men are beginning to want to be known, to be seen. There is a power in being known and seen, but it is not power as men traditionally understand it. Being known is a vulnerable position; it also makes communication possible. For this reason modern penis art carries cultural significance. It signifies the dismantling of a barrier, the opening of a door.

SELECTED PENIS ARTISTS

Many of the artists whose work includes penises and erections are homosexual men. For them the penis, the erection, the nude male body are objects of desire—and objects that they have not been allowed to show. When in the 1970s Robert Mapplethorpe began photographing naked male bodies or parts of bodies, often engaged in so-called transgressive sexual acts, it was not only an aesthetic choice but a political act. Formally his photographs are exquisite; the combination of elegance of eye with sexually explosive content is what makes his work both glamorous and important.

In his many photographs with the same title, *Cock*, penises are sometimes used as a design element, seen as the center and root of the man, thrusting out between dark, mysterious legs; or they're in close-up, partially bound in leather, so the cock skin looks supple and luscious. *Man in Polyester Suit* presents a suit-wearing male torso. The lines of the suit are boxy and straight-edged; everything is neat except that the fly is open, and a huge cock descends, like a tongue hanging out. Formally, the organic works against the manufactured. And the image has the wit of a wish fulfilled; it's what almost everyone really wants to know.

At the same time Mapplethorpe was working, Keith Haring was putting dicks all over his paintings. Because the paintings were deliberately childlike, and the images were of animals and children, no one thought to object to the phallic content.

Andy Warhol, going Renoir one better, sometimes mixed urine or semen with his paints, or literally painted with his prick. He also gave us the grainy black-and-white film *Blow Job,* which for thirty-five minutes concentrates on a man's face as he gets fellated off camera.

Another reason for the current focus on penises is a pervasive interest in the body as both source and subject of art. For heterosexual male artists, working with erect penises is a bold way of looking at sexuality. Andres Serrano's 1997 New York show, called *A History of Sex,* consisted of beautifully composed large color photographs of outrageous couples—an old woman and a young man, a big man and a pretty girl dwarf, a woman and a horse— in bucolic settings. Whatever these people may be doing —or about to do—their expressions are so serene, and they look like such nice people, that viewers are challenged to ask themselves, Why not? Someone holding his own quite large erection, who's outdoors with blue sky and water behind him, who's looking off pensively into the middle distance, a smile playing about his lips as if he's thinking about something funny his accountant just told him, brings the erection into the realm of images you can examine closely, and even discuss with your accountant.

Women artists have also been working with penis imagery, and for them it's not only a way of expanding the vocabulary of images we can see and talk about, it's also a way of confronting, or sending up, men. One early example (1974) is the "ad" Lynda Benglis placed in *Art Forum,* a full-page color photograph of herself wearing dark glasses and nothing else except a long, erect dildo protruding from between her legs. No words were needed.

Recently I visited Rhonda Shearer, who was preparing an interactive show with a penis motif. She wanted to play, she said, with our fears about looking at genitalia in art and life. Among the works was a mannequin of a little girl in a pretty pink dress with a big rubber dick under her skirt. There was also a wall with eighty-nine mostly very big talking dildos on it, which Shearer calls the Tunnel. The show's fun-house atmosphere makes prejudices against genitals into a joke—but Shearer told me men found the Tunnel intimidating. "When they realize that all of a sudden they're the sex object they tend to get quiet, or more introspective. It's an interesting turn," she said.

TWO ARTISTS WHOSE SUBJECT IS DICKS

TOM OF FINLAND

Anyone who's interested in penis art should know about Tom of Finland (1920–1991), the originator of the erotic drawing style seen in today's gay pinup magazines. Tom drew men's men—lumberjacks, cowboys, soldiers, sailors, bikers—anyone who could wear a uniform and very tight pants. You could see their enormous cocks outlined by the pants or, sometimes, out sailing in the breeze.

Lucky Tom always drew with a hard-on. His biographer, F. Valentine Hooven III, quotes him: "I knew who the boss was—my cock. It did not matter how much my head liked an idea—or, in later years, how much money I was promised; if my cock did not stand up while I was working on a drawing, I could not make the drawing work."

In addition to his boldness in depicting dicks, Tom's good nature is obvious in the drawings. The men are enjoying each other. He once said, "I wouldn't mind being known as the Norman Rockwell of gay erotica." His first published drawing was in the spring 1957 issue of *Physique Pictorial*, which was the way gay men in those days got their pinups. Eventually his work was shown at the Whitney Museum and sold at Christie's.

Tom said of all the huge penises he drew: "Cock size doesn't matter to me. I didn't start doing those giant cocks until the censors let the magazines publish full frontal nudity. I had to come up with *something* you couldn't get in a photograph."

CYNTHIA PLASTER CASTER

Cynthia Plaster Caster started in the 1960s as a Chicago groupie whose gimmick was, with various assistants, to make plaster casts of the cocks of rock musicians. In 1968 *Rolling Stone* published an issue on groupies with a page devoted to Cynthia and her crew, and they spoke of their methods. One of them performed fellatio (they called the activity "plating") on the prospective penis, and when it was properly hard the other had the materials ready. Sometimes they were too stoned to do it right, or something went wrong technically, or the guy's erection wilted when he was asked to plunge it into a malt shaker full of Caulk Fast Set. That's the same material dentists use, Cynthia told me, "the pink stuff they put in your mouth to take impressions of your teeth and gums."

Currently Cynthia's cock casts, some in bronze, some in white plaster, number in the forties. "Sometimes I've only captured half a shaft or just a head of somebody, and that's not to say that's all they had to offer; that's all I was able to capture with my inept, amateur-style casting. Some of them actually look like pigs' tails or little corkscrews. They were unfortunately going soft in that fashion just as the mold was hardening."

The first twenty-two or so were done before 1971 and include Jimi Hendrix, Noel Redding and Zal Yanofsky of the Lovin' Spoonful. Between 1971 and 1980 she didn't capture anyone. "I just didn't care for the music in the seventies, and the sexual revolution was taking a down-swing—it wasn't fashionable to be trying different kinds of sex out or dipping your dick into something new and different." Now, she says, "There are more people inter-ested than there ever were—of the type I would be inter-ested in casting."

The longest cock in her collection is "probably Clint Poppie, lead singer of the Dead Kennedys. He's one of the curved ones. You have to be kind of long to curve." And Jimi Hendrix? "It was really thick. If I were to curl my fore-finger and thumb around it they would be about an inch apart. I remember him being on the long side, too. But I wasn't in on the stimulation for that one. It was my plater who was choking on that."

MORE FAMOUS PENISES IN ART

It would be impossible, within the scope of this book, to present a full array of twentieth-century artists who've worked with penises. The following are some, not previously mentioned at any length, whose work I saw or heard about while I was doing my research.

FORERUNNERS:

Thomas Eakins—The famous nineteenth-century Philadelphia realist painter of domestic and sporting scenes also photographed naked young men, some of them his students.

Baron Wilhelm von Gloeden—German photographer moved to Sicily in the late nineteenth century, where he photographed sunlit naked youth in classical poses, sometimes wearing laurel wreaths.

Paul Cadmus—the grand old man of twentieth-century homoerotic art; became famous for *The Fleet's In!* (1934), a painting of sailors carousing with streetwalkers that the navy found objectionably sordid. In this as in his other work, the men's clothing is so tight their crotches bulge. One man, offering a sailor a light, wears a bright red tie, a coded symbol for homosexuality.

SURREALISTS:

Pierre Molinier—French surrealist photographed himself in wigs, corsets and black fishnet stockings, sometimes with his penis showing, sometimes with a homemade dildo covering his genitals. These dildos might also be placed, for purposes of masturbation, on the backs of his high-heeled shoes.

Jindrich Styrsky—Czech surrealist in 1933 privately published a book of erotic photo-collage dream images, *Emilie Comes to Me in a Dream*. Penises—and vaginas—predominated.

THE SIXTIES:

Carolee Schneemann—body artist; first publicly used the penis in 1965 in *Fuses*, a self-shot eighteen-minute,

16mm film in which she makes love with her partner—paying particular attention to his erect and glistening prick.

Larry Rivers—uses penises whenever suitable. His 1969 relief *America's No. 1 Problem* consisted of two penises on silver Mylar, one dark brown, one pink, both exactly nine inches long, according to the ruler at the bottom of the picture.

Yayoi Kusama—covered a variety of everyday objects with painted, stuffed, cloth penises—sofa, chair, ironing board, rowboat, etc. She said she worked with penises because they scared her.

Vito Acconci—In his performance piece *Seedbed*, 1972, he masturbated, unseen, beneath a specially built ramp in the Sonnabend Gallery. Visitors would walk on the ramp and listen for the sounds of ecstasy coming from below.

Judith Bernstein—showed enormous, intense charcoal drawings of hairy screws—some horizontal, some vertical—that looked suspiciously like erections.

THE NINETIES:

Francesco Clemente—His drawings and paintings are often erotic, and include erect penises as a matter of course.

Gilbert and George—in 1997 did a show of enlarged photographs of their own excretions seen under a microscope—*Spunk Blood Piss Shit Spit* is one of the titles—with the two of them, naked, wandering through all the fluids.

Cecily Brown—in 1998 showed canvases full of thrusting Technicolor erections; the paintings are named for movie musicals—*High Society, Seven Brides for Seven Brothers*, etc.

Matthias Herrmann—German photographer takes nude self-portraits, many of them close-ups of his erections, some of them lit in luscious Popsicle colors.

Carroll Dunham—paints cartoon figures of fighting men, usually perched around the edges of some geometric form, wielding knives, guns and dynamite sticks. Cocks that protrude from their heads or bellies aim pellets of come at each other.

Paul McCarthy—This bad-boy performance artist uses penises in drawings and sculptures, live and on video, and has been seen, in performance, covering his own penis with mustard and ketchup, treating it like a hot dog.

Steven Haas—photographs flaccid penises in black-and-white close-up so they look like lush, immaculate still lifes of leeks and eggplants.

CHAPTER

FIVE

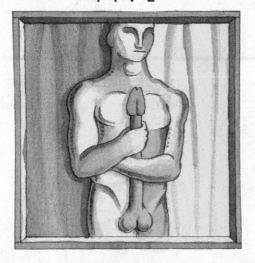

MOVIE
PENISES

Anyone who watches Hollywood movies knows they rarely allow for visible penises. You can hardly see a realistic sex scene in a Hollywood movie, never mind full frontal male nudity. When there is a frontally nude male he's generally not a big star and the shot is fleeting; he's not expected to act with his penis hanging out. The fearless Harvey Keitel, an actor who wants to expand the boundaries of what's permissible, is the exception who proves the rule. After all, why shouldn't Robert Redford keep his clothes on and leave well enough alone? As illustrator Robert Richards said to me, "It's going to be a very long time before we ever see mainstream male stars revealing themselves. And that's because of the penis. Because they sell themselves as supervirile, magic-god people, these stars. There's almost no point in going to a Kevin Costner movie or a Robert Redford movie because their characters are so defined—they're always up to making love; they're also up to saving nations, to derailing trains, to changing the way we think. They're so heroic, and somehow that makes up for nudity, and that becomes their penis. The superheroic character that they've created is a penis. For any of these stars to show a real penis would be a big anticlimax."

PENIS MOVIES

A few brave filmmakers have tried, with varying degrees of success, to acknowledge the penis. These are some of their movies:

Marquis, 1990, conceived by Roland Topor, directed by Henri Xhonneux. A French movie based on the writings of the Marquis de Sade, was set in the Bastille in 1789 and performed by people wearing animal heads. Justine is a cow, Juliette is a horse, the captain of the Bastille is a rooster, the prison guard is a rat, the Marquis is a dog, and he has an extremely large and animated prosthetic talking penis with a handsome and sensitive human face. The penis and the Marquis engage in long conversations about who rules whom. The Marquis is melancholy; the penis, whom he calls Colin, is mischievous and outspoken. He'll tell the Marquis, "I need exercise," or he'll say, "You're not the boss. I can make you lose your head." In the end they escape from prison, and Colin leaves the Marquis for Juliette. The Marquis bends resignedly over his writings. "Not too many verbs, now," Colin says.

In the Realm of the Senses, 1976, directed by Nagisa Oshima. This extremely erotic Japanese movie, based on a true story and set in 1936, is about a man and a woman, Kichi-san and Sada, who become so sexually obsessed with each other they can't stop doing it, over and over again. When they're not naked with each other, Kichi-san is lifting the skirt of Sada's kimono, or she's parting the entrance to his. Neither of them wears underwear. Sada adores Kichi-san's beautiful purple penis. At one of the geisha houses they stay in together the proprietress tells her, "The geishas won't come in, they say you're disgusting. You do nothing but suck him all day long." "That's not disgusting," Sada says. But in the end she's too possessive—she wants to kill Kichi-san so he'll never put himself inside another woman. He's so exhausted he says, "Do what you please, my body is yours forever." With his consent she strangles him while they're fucking. Then she cuts off his cock with a kitchen knife and lies beside him, organ in hand. Screen titles tell us the real Sada wandered around Tokyo for four days, holding her severed penis and glowing with happiness, before she was apprehended.

During the 1970s, when the sexual revolution was in flower, the British produced several comedies revolving around penises. *Percy,* 1971, directed by Ralph Thomas, is about a man who receives the first penis transplant and finds out what he can about its previous owner. *It's Not the Size That Counts,* 1974, is about the same man, this time played by a different actor. *The Statue,* 1971, directed by Rod Amateau and starring David Niven, is about a twenty-foot statue of Niven that sports an enormous dick. These films are all so bad that most video stores don't carry them.

In the late 1990s, films began to find new uses for the penis. *The Full Monty* (1997), directed by Peter Cattaneo, is about out-of-work British laborers who create their own strip show, exhibiting their penises for money though we, the movie audience, never see them. A penis appears at the end of *Boogie Nights,* Paul Thomas Anderson's 1997 movie about the X-rated film and video industry, when the great porn star, played by Mark Wahlberg, faces a mirror to look at himself in all his glory. The penis seen on-screen is a very large prosthetic device, as false as the enormous nose an actor must wear if he wants to play Cyrano de Bergerac.

X-RATED VIDEOS

Hollywood may be shy about showing full frontal male nudity, but that doesn't mean Americans never see penises on-screen. To the contrary. We make up for what we don't see at the movies by watching X-rated videos at home. In fact, almost a quarter of the revenue of the multibillion-dollar home video market comes from rentals and sales of X-rated videos. The majority of these videos are good-natured bacchanals, in which the sexual performances are meant to remind viewers that they could be doing something similar. Since most of the videos are made with men in mind, their principal subject is the adventures of the penis—as it labors to get in and out of as many locations as possible, as often as possible in the allotted time.

I rented the following X-rated videos—two heterosexuals, one homosexual—as part of my fieldwork.

1) *Rocco More Than Ever.* The clerk at the video store told me gay men like videos by the Italian porn star Rocco —even though there's no sex between men—because of the size of Rocco's cock. Rocco's cock—which is big, fat and juicy-looking—and the similar but redder cock of the actor who in this video plays his pal, Giovanni, are the stars of the show. There isn't much plot. We meet the men outside of Buckingham Palace, looking for women to film

having sex with them. They start with a woman they pick up during the changing of the guard, and end at an English country house full of women and men who have sex with each other all day long. Rocco's handheld camera gives the video an intimate, documentary look. As in most contemporary films, there are subplots. Just as you're tiring of the barnyard scene—with the dominatrix, the woman who services her, the black groom who also services her, the indefatigable Giovanni, and a tethered horse—you're switched back to the bedroom, where the skinny blonde is having anal sex with Rocco and vaginal sex with her boyfriend Chris at the same time. Her teddy bear watches, its strap-on dildo erect and ready.

2) *All About Eva*. Like *All About Eve*, the X-rated version begins and ends at an awards ceremony where a great new star is being honored—but there the resemblance ends. Unlike Eve, who was a scheming actress, Eva betrays her way to the top of the world of adult entertainment. Most of the video is a flashback to a porn-star party where, instead of engaging in repartee, the characters take off their clothes and get inside each other.

3) *Stryker Force* stars the boyishly handsome Jeff Stryker and the big, strong and ever-ready penis that made him famous. Its plot takes Jeff and five other men—some friends, some rivals—into a jungle to look for buried treasure. There they tramp around shirtless, displaying admirably developed abs, pecs and delts. As soon as they stop walking they begin having sex. Jeff's tall, graceful dick stands up like a tree when he's lying down.

Someone who was learning about human mating habits by watching these videos would have to conclude that penises either taste very good or have curative properties that can be absorbed through the tongue. As soon as Mr. Friendly emerges from its protective trousers, someone

73

always pounces on it, taking it into his or her mouth. Suffering obvious discomfort to neck, mouth and throat, this lucky individual then pumps up and down on the shaft until it gets taken away and placed in some other venue.

An erect penis causes frenzied activity among those in its vicinity. This is seen most clearly in fast-forward mode. Penises keep thrusting, thrusting, thrusting, as the partners change positions and orifices and more people with penises and orifices get added to the mix. In fact, the partners seem to be going through the routines of a thorough cleaning, with the kind of care you might take to make sure the silver got polished on all sides: front to front, front to back, side to side, head to tail, head to head.

At the end of each sequence the penis pulls out of its burrow so it can erupt on camera, spraying semen. Sometimes it points and aims its load, usually at a participating woman. Sometimes it's whipped around, and the flecks fly all over. In the Italian video a woman always gets semen in the face; she licks it off hungrily, as if it were chocolate sauce.

Enrique came over while I was in the middle of *Stryker Force* and saw the conclusion with me. He thought it was boring and the acting was wooden. "It's like ice-skating," he said. "They perform all these wonderful physical feats but the people have no expression. You don't care about them."

I had to remind him that just like watching X-rated videos, watching ice-skating on TV is an increasingly popular American pastime.

CHAPTER

SIX

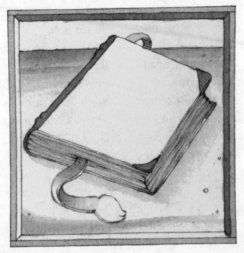

PENIS LANGUAGE AND LITERATURE

There once was a young man from Kent
Whose thing was so long that it bent.
To save himself trouble
He put it in double,
And instead of coming he went.

LANGUAGE

It's taken three hundred years for penis, the word, to enter the English vernacular. Penis, Latin for tail, was first employed in English in a late-seventeenth-century medical text—and because it sounds scientific it gained limited currency as a euphemism when the commonly used "prick" began to seem too racy. But it never really caught on, probably because it was meant for polite conversations, and no one wanted to have polite conversations about pricks. At least not until recently.

Ever since penis became a word of choice for the 1990s it's been a regular feature in books and movies, where characters use it to have polite conversations about pricks. These conversations hardly existed in books and movies before. In movies penises just weren't mentioned. In books, for sexual descriptions, writers usually preferred more intimate, sexy words like cock and prick—the words actual lovers use.

Use of the word penis has brought the word dick along with it almost into the mainstream. Penis is a more formal word than dick. With the word penis you can have a casual conversation in a restaurant, even with your mother, if she's game. Use the word dick and your mother might think you were taking liberties. Dick is a better word for telling jokes with—but the word penis, because it's awkward to say, and it conjures up something anatomically ungainly, can itself be used for comic effect. Though dick can't be used on television or in a family newspaper, it's preferred in some books and movies—for example, the movie *Chasing Amy,* about a love affair between a heterosexual man and a woman who's a lesbian most of the time. These characters pride themselves on their frankness about sex, and the companionable dick is the best word for that frankness.

There are many other words that can be used to mean penis, and if you search you can find lists of them. On the Internet there's an erection page, where the proprietor hopes to collect "the world's largest (no pun intended) collection of names for an erection." The annual readers' survey in a magazine called *Men* includes a list sent in by readers. Such lists overflow with fanciful, affectionate names like "bald-headed mouse," "love rod" and "husband of nature," which people must stay up late at night inventing.

In China and India the penis is addressed with deference: Indian/Tibetan terms include Arrow of Love, Jewel, Scepter; among the Chinese terms are Jade Stalk, Jade Flute, Crimson Bird, Ambassador.

The common English words for penis, on the other hand, are likely to be disrespectful: dick, prick, cock, schlong, joint, Johnson, meat, member, pecker, rod, peter, putz, tool, willy, dong, wong, ding-dong, weenie ("family jewels" would seem to be an exception, but I've never heard it used without irony). Rude terms for an erection include: boner, hard-on, woody, pecker wood, chubby, stiffy. In New Zealand, I was told, getting a hard-on is called "snarling," because "it's angry and it's just about to bite you."

In America we sometimes use words for the penis in describing people. These terms are never complimentary. A prick is a mean, hard penis or person; a dick is friendly but pushy, at the ready, maybe not too bright; a putz is little and mean; a schlong is big and sloppy; a pecker is hard and wily; a tool is just a tool; a dickhead is totally annoying and stupid; a cocksucker is the lowest of the low. (Right here you have the essence of men's ambivalence about their cocks. They love having them sucked, and yet they find it unthinkable that anyone—particularly anyone male—could love to suck them.)

Joint and rod are businesslike appellations, and we don't apply them to people. A ding-dong is an idiot, someone who has no control over his private parts or anything else. I like the term Johnson for a penis, because of its dignity and formality. Roger is another man's name that can mean penis; to roger also means to fuck. Etymologists think roger came to be used for penis because farmers in the seventeenth and eighteenth centuries for some reason used to give the name to their bulls.

Prick and cock are two of the oldest English names for the penis. Shakespeare used prick to mean penis in the sixteenth century in such punning verses as this from *As You Like It*: "He that sweetest rose will find/Must find love's prick and Rosalinde." During the sixteenth and early seventeenth centuries prick was even used as a pet name, but by the late seventeenth century prudery had set in, and the word was gradually banned from written language. In 1861, bowdlerizers changed the above passage from *As You Like It* to read, "Must find love's *thorn* and Rosalinde." The first use of prick as a name for a penislike person was dated to 1929 by the *Oxford English Dictionary,* but lexicographer Hugh Rawson, to whose *Wicked Words* I'm indebted for this account, believes the usage is much older.

Cock derives from the word for the male barnyard fowl, and is such a common synonym for penis that two hundred years ago prudish Americans began referring to that fowl as a rooster. A number of other words were changed in the late eighteenth and early nineteenth centuries to appease offended sensibilities. Apricock became apricot; haycock became haystack; weathercock became weathervane.

Schlong is Yiddish for snake, or penis. Putz and schmuck are rude Yiddish terms for penis that derive from German words for ornament or jewel. Putz is worse than schmuck. Both are now used almost entirely to mean jerk. Yet as recently as 1962 the groundbreaking comic Lenny Bruce was arrested in Los Angeles for using schmuck and putz on stage—"by a Yiddish undercover agent," Bruce said in *How to Talk Dirty and Influence People,* "who had been placed in the club several nights running to determine if my use of Yiddish terms was a cover for profanity." For elderly Jews the terms are still taboo.

Dick meaning penis dates back at least to 1891. The term may derive from Donkey Dick, which was what people used to call male jackasses in the eighteenth century. In the American underworld a dick is a detective and a policewoman is a Dickless Tracy. Dick is also used as a verb, meaning to copulate or to cheat—as in this piece of graffiti cited in *American Speech* in 1980, "Dick Nixon before he dicks you."

LITERATURE

Penises have adorned our songs and stories for as long as songs and stories have existed. Shakespeare's plays were strewn with double entendres involving pricks and cocks. Rabelais, in the rambunctious *Gargantua and Pantagruel,* brought up penises whenever the spirit took him; the Marquis de Sade wrote about little else. But it wasn't until D. H. Lawrence published his erotic masterpiece, *Lady Chatterley's Lover,* that descriptions of sex acts in plain English became part of literature. First printed in an edition of 1,000 copies in Italy in 1928, *Lady Chatterley's Lover* created a sensation even though most people had to read an expurgated version, missing all the sensational parts. It became a milestone in the fight against censorship when the entire text was published in New York in 1959 and a U.S. District Court judge ruled that it was not obscene.

Liberated by that decision, fiction writers in the U.S. and Britain have published innumerable descriptions of sex acts and penises performing them. In at least four of these works, penises have attained the status of memorable characters. If you read the works in chronological order

79

you can observe the way our attitudes toward penises have changed.

MEMORABLE PENISES IN LITERATURE

LADY CHATTERLEY'S LOVER

D. H. Lawrence, an enemy of industrialization, believed in the redeeming power of natural impulses—which could be activated by lusty, uninhibited sex. The penis was essential to the plan. In *Lady Chatterley's Lover* Lawrence was rhapsodic about the penis. His descriptions of its charms and powers, which today seem a bit overexcited, were then quite shocking and took courage to write.

Connie Chatterley, the heroine, is in trouble when her effete husband Clifford, injured in the First World War, returns home wheelchair-bound and impotent. Friends of Clifford's visit the estate, and he makes it clear he wouldn't mind Connie having an affair. Connie tries one of Clifford's friends—but she falls in love with Mellors, the gamekeeper. Mellors is a natural man, not a priss, an intellectual or a poof. Connie always used to have her orgasm after the man's, doing it for herself, using his penis. With Mellors she surrenders; she lets him lead, she lets passion take her.

Mellors calls his penis John Thomas, and although he speaks good English, when he speaks to John Thomas he uses the local dialect he spoke as a child. "Tha ma'es nowt o me, John Thomas," he says. "Art boss? of me? Eh well, tha'rt more cocky than me, an' tha says less. John Thomas! Dost want *her*? Dost want my lady Jane?"

"So proud," Connie says of it (or him). "And so lordly! Now I know why men are so overbearing. But he's lovely, *really*. Like another being! A bit terrifying! But lovely really!" Connie braids forget-me-nots into Mellors's pubic hair. He does the same to her, then winds creeping Jennie vine around John Thomas.

Lawrence's total faith in the phallus may be old-fashioned—but even by today's standards *Lady Chatterley* is compellingly straightforward about sex and relations between the sexes. Here he describes the carnal and spiritual passion of deep sexual love: "In the short summer night she learnt so much. She would have thought a woman would have died of shame. Instead of which, the shame died. Shame, which is fear: the deep organic shame, the old, old physical fear which crouches in the bodily roots of us, and can only be chased away by the sensual fire, at last it was rouse up [*sic*] and routed by the phallic hunt of the man, and she came to the very heart of the jungle of herself. . . . So! That was how it was! That was life; That was how oneself really was! There was nothing left to disguise or be ashamed of. She shared her ultimate nakedness with a man, another being."

THE TIME OF HER TIME

In *Lady Chatterley's Lover* Lawrence celebrated the wonders of cock, totally without irony. But by the time that novel came to the U.S. the balance of power between the sexes had shifted. Norman Mailer's story "The Time of Her Time," published in *Advertisements for Myself* (1961), was also famous for phallic bravado, yet its hero, Sergius O'Shaughnessy, is filled with discontent. Sergius calls his penis the avenger, in that half-serious, half-mocking way that Mailer has. The story begins when Sergius meets a young, aggressive Jewish woman who says she's never had an orgasm. He hardly even likes the woman, but he wants to be the one to make her come, so she'll never forget him.

He fucks her on three separate nights, subjecting the avenger to a beating. Finally he pushes her over the edge by penetrating her anally—and for good measure calling her a dirty Jew. He thinks they've won, he and the avenger, but then she trumps him. She says her analyst warned her Sergius was a repressed homosexual, and what he just did proves it. As she walks out he realizes, too late, that this was a woman worthy of him.

PORTNOY'S COMPLAINT

Lady Chatterley's Lover and "The Time of Her Time" are romantic tales about the penis and its power in the world. In Philip Roth's *Portnoy's Complaint,* published in 1969, the penis is a comic character, and it's driving the hero crazy. Alternately adored and smothered by his terror of a Jewish mother, Portnoy would be the kind of man his mother wants him to be if it weren't for his penis. He wants to be good, but his penis loves trouble, and it demands his constant attention. He addresses his story to his therapist. Here's a small sample: "Then came adolescence —half my waking life spent locked behind the bathroom door, firing my wad down the toilet bowl, or into the soiled clothes in the laundry hamper, or *splat,* up against the medicine-chest mirror, before which I stood in my dropped drawers so I could see how it looked coming out. Or else I was doubled over my flying fist, eyes pressed closed but mouth wide open, to take that sticky sauce of buttermilk and Clorox on my own tongue and teeth— though not infrequently, in my blindness and ecstasy, I got it all in the pompadour, like a blast of Wildroot Cream Oil."

Most famously he masturbates with raw liver—"rolled round my cock in the bathroom at three-thirty—and then had again on the end of a fork, at five-thirty, along with the other member of that poor innocent family of mine.

"So. Now you know the worst thing I have ever done. I fucked my own family's dinner."

COCK & BULL

Will Self's two comic novellas are about a woman whose clitoris becomes a penis, and a man who grows a vagina behind one of his knees. In *Cock*, the one that matters for our purposes, the protagonist, Carol, becomes more matter-of-fact, practical and assertive as her cock grows bigger. Once she's full-grown she rapes her husband. And acquires a taste for violating others.

Cock & Bull got well reviewed but it didn't cause the same kind of stir as its three predecessors. By the time it was published, in the early 1990s, readers had grown a bit blasé.

By the late 1990s, in New York at least, you could ask your studious-looking neighborhood librarian for help in researching penises and he wouldn't even flinch.

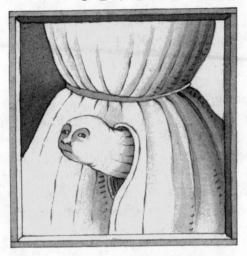

THE PENIS
IN FASHION

A t first glance penises would seem to be totally irrelevant to fashion. Not glamorous enough for evenings, too obtrusive for office wear. But in other times and places men have dressed with their penises in mind. Some do the same in the U.S. in the late 1990s—and others might like to.

THINGS MEN WEAR THAT DRAW ATTENTION TO THEIR DICKS

NOTHING BUT A KYNODESME

In Classical Greece, young men exercised—and often walked around—in the nude. To protect his penis from wear and tear, a man would pull the tip of his foreskin over his glans and tie it together with a ribbon or a leather string. Then, so they wouldn't flap, he'd knot the ends of the string around the base of his penis. The whole thing made a pretty little bundle that was called a *kynodesme*, or dog knot. According to *The Reign of the Phallus*, "The dog knot was the ancient equivalent of the modern jock strap and, like that item of men's clothing, acquired associations of male sexual pride and supremacy."

CODPIECES

During the late Middle Ages and early Renaissance in Europe men began wearing clothes that emphasized their penises. It started in the fourteenth century; coats and tights were the fashion, and then coats got short. By 1360 coats only reached mid-thigh, and when a man sat down, or bent over, anyone could see the shape of his genitals through his tights. To cover their dicks, men moved their money pouches from the side, where they used to hang, to the front. But these pouches were brightly colored and only drew attention to the area; to add to the effect the men wore their daggers and swords behind their pouches, dangling suggestively between their legs. Dressing this way was popular. An English law forbidding the practice to anyone under the rank of lord, esquire or gentleman went unobserved, and had to be proclaimed again and again.

Then, during the fifteenth century, the codpiece became the height of fashion. Codpieces were padded pouches for the cock and balls, gaily colored and meant to be seen. Some were shaped like penises with erections that pointed straight up. Others were more fanciful. In Bronzino's *Portrait of Lodovico Capponi* at the Frick Collection in New York, the codpiece peeks out from beneath the elegant young man's jacket, round and ridged like an eager piece of upholstery. Codpieces also functioned as purses—men used them to carry coins, sweets and handkerchiefs.

Some fashion historians think codpieces were invented to cover the genitals under short coats. But their original purpose may have been to protect expensive fabrics from the stains of mercury-based syphilis creams. Or they may have started out as pieces of armor, when armor switched from chain mail to riveted metal plates. In photographs of armor of the period, for example Henry VIII's Greenwich armor for the field and tilt, 1540, the codpiece juts out from between the legs, snub-nosed and almost as wide as a forearm, like a small, shiny battering ram.

(Apparently, during the period when young knights were wearing codpieces, monks were walking around naked under their skirts. Here's the opinion of François Rabelais—who was himself a monk before leaving the convent to study medicine—from his great *Gargantua and Pantagruel*: "'. . . what makes the tools of the poor blessed fathers so long is that they do not wear bottomed breeches, and their poor member stretches freely, without let or hindrance, and so it goes waggling down to their knees, like a woman's string of beads. But the reason why they have it correspondingly stout is because as it waggles the humours of the body descend into the said member. For according to the lawmen, agitation and continual motion are the cause of attraction.'")

Codpieces sound like a fashion men could love. Dealing with a heftily padded symbolic erection all day long must have made them feel perpetually aroused. Probably there were competitions over who had the biggest and the prettiest. But if you were a woman you might, after a while, begin to tire of thrusting phalluses. Whatever the reason, by the end of the sixteenth century the codpiece went out of fashion. By the end of the seventeenth century the word "cod"—which had originally meant scrotum, and later meant pouch, or bag—had come to mean fool.

Even today men might love codpieces, if someone revived them in the right way. If we had codpieces today, with our advanced technology, they could look like anything a man wanted: a police car, a Scud missile, a pit bull, a submarine, a submarine sandwich, an Academy Award —or even, if the wearer were really out there, an anatomically correct monster erection.

In the late 1970s Eldridge Cleaver—the former Black Panther, famous in the '60s as the author of *Soul on Ice*— tried reviving codpieces, but he was probably too political about it. In *Jet* magazine Cleaver said that the penis was covered up in modern dress because its visibility would have "a slowing down effect on efficiency and production." He said men had been "castrated" by pants, and he intended to reverse the trend by manufacturing and selling "Cleavers," trousers with codpiece built in. There were two types of codpieces—one was shaped like a football player's oval jockey cup, the other like a cock and balls. Cleaver invested $42,000 of his own money in a small pants factory and a retail store in West Hollywood; it was a bad career move on his part.

PENIS SHEATHS

For many men in primitive cultures, the proper way to dress up a penis is with a decorative sheath. As of 1969, penis sheaths were still being worn in Africa, South America, New Guinea and the Southwest Pacific Islands, sometimes by men who wore nothing else.

Sheaths vary widely in size and shape. All of them cover the head of the penis, some being little more than caps, and most of them cover the shaft as well. In some cultures a man's sheath indicates his status; often a boy is given his first sheath with his initiation rites. Some cultures have everyday sheaths, festival sheaths, war-going sheaths; in some the men only wear sheaths on certain occasions and otherwise go naked. In some the sheath-wearing seems to be a fashion statement. According to the anthropologist Peter J. Ucko, whose 1969 lecture "Penis Sheaths: A Comparative Study" is the authoritative resource in the field, ". . . the Bafia of the Cameroons . . . wear a multiplicity of sheath forms each with its own distinctive name. New styles of sheaths are continually being introduced and, once approved, are quickly copied by others. Any Bafia can make his own normal, everyday, sheath from strips of palm leaves . . . only specialist Bafia can make the type of leaf sheath which has two points . . . Only certain master craftsmen amongst the Bafia can make certain rare types of sheaths and those worn during festivals, all of which are covered with snake or lizard skin and are characterised by their rounded off corners and the use of decorative sewing, colouring and the sophisticated inclusion of decorative additions such as feathers and claws."

Sheaths may be made out of braided vegetable fibers, gourds, shells, bamboo, aluminum, cocoons, ivory, coconut, skin, leather, horn. Gourd sheaths are often shaped while still on the vine. "Amongst the Dani of New Guinea a long and straight gourd is obtained by attaching a stone weight to the growing gourd; a curved or curving gourd results from bending and lashing it while growing," and so on. When they're ready they're roasted and scraped on the outside and the meat inside is scooped out and then they may be sun-dried to bring out their yellow color.

In some societies like the Kapauku, a man owns his sheath and never lends it. In others, like the Dani, every man has a big sheath wardrobe, including some suitable to give to visitors.

In some societies the penis, sheathed or not, is held in an erect position with the aid of a hip or waist belt. Some hold the sheath upright with a rope around the neck or under the armpits. A documentary about a tribe who rope their sheaths was aired recently. The sheaths looked like long, straight poles, rooted at the penis and poking straight up to shoulder height. When a man bent to hoe the garden his sheath bounced in front of him, obstructing his view. When he climbed trees and wove branches together to build a bridge he had to push his own branch out of his way. Members of this tribe must learn to give each other a wide berth, or risk having an eye poked out.

Sheaths aren't necessarily easy to get on. Several peoples in New Guinea use a kind of spatula made from a pig's tusk to ease the penis into its sheath, "more or less as a shoe horn is used in Europe today: the spatula, being considered an essential accessory to the sheath, is worn in the hair for easy accessibility." Once the sheath is in place it's likely to irritate the penis inside; loose-fitting sheaths often fall off; if the fit is firm a man can't have an erection while wearing his sheath.

Anthropologists know that penis sheaths are important in tribal life, but they don't know why, exactly. A sheath covers the penis, hiding it from prying eyes and protecting it from both wear and tear and evil spirits. On the other hand it draws attention to the penis and its reputed magical powers. It functions as a constant symbol of an erection, yet it may prevent a man from having an erection. Some think it gives a man the penis he wishes he had. In any case it clarifies the question of who's a man and who isn't.

JAPANESE PENIS PACKAGING

Japan is a country that values packaging, and by the eighth century some Shinto priests there had invented a way to package penises. Kokigami, the art of penis packaging, is designed to heighten the pleasure of sex. This art reached its height in Japan in the ninth to twelfth centuries, and is practiced today by those who are so inclined. The man packs his penis inside a paper sculpture of an animal; once the sculpture is in place he can imagine his penis has the qualities of the animal, and he and his partner can act out sexual fantasies the animal inspires. Scripts are available, if desired, to guide the fantasies. A slang term for Kokigami is "the Nippon slip-on."

PHALLIC SYMBOLS IN FASHION

From the late eleventh until the late fifteenth century in Europe, long, pointed shoes called *poulaines* were in vogue. They were invented by Norman knights to give feet a better fit inside stirrups. But walking in them couldn't have been easy, and their continuing popularity was probably related to the widely accepted idea that foot size reflected penis size. For a while it was the fashion for the long tips to be filled with sawdust so they stood upright. Apparently some *poulaine* wearers shaped and colored the extension to emphasize its resemblance to a penis. Charles V of France prohibited the wearing of penis-shaped *poulaines* in 1367.

Hats are also considered by fashion historians to be misplaced penises. James Laver makes the point, in *Modesty in Dress*, that during the nineteenth century in England, men's hats decreased in height in proportion to the rise of feminine emancipation. By the century's end they were wearing, "so to speak, the very symbol of their bashed-in authority: the trilby [a soft-brimmed felt hat with a bashed-in crown]."

A tie is an obvious phallic symbol, when you think about it. It hangs there, looking good, the only rakish part of a modern businessman's outfit. Men pay attention to selecting their ties, which, along with shirts, are their principle source of decoration. In novelty stores you can buy a tie that's flesh-colored and has a dick its own size painted on it.

SUITS

For the past century and a half the suit has been the male uniform, concealing the penis behind a pair of trousers, and over that a jacket. The penis may be hidden, but everyone still knows it's there—covering it up merely shows it doesn't need to be seen in order to be felt. Anne Hollander, in *Sex and Suits*, defines the suit mentality as "the enduring conception that men's clothes are honest, comfortable and utilitarian, whereas women's are difficult, deceptive and foolish."

A man habitually wears his penis against one leg or the other, and this is known as "dressing" to the right or the left. Whichever side he dresses on, his penis, under loose-fitting twentieth-century trousers, is easily within his reach. Given the opportunity, some men masturbate by putting their hands in their trouser pockets and grabbing their cocks without anyone being the wiser. This practice is known as "pocket pool."

ROCK & ROLL

The 1960s were a good time for penises. Tight pants, which hadn't been fashionable for men since the first half of the nineteenth century, returned as rock-star regalia— and rock stars didn't just wear their pants skin-tight, they routinely stuffed them to accentuate the bulge in the crotch. In fact, bulging jeans became a rock & roll joke. One of the most famous images in rock & roll is Andy Warhol's sleeve for the Rolling Stones album *Sticky Fingers*. It's a black-and-white photograph of the jeans-clad crotch of Warhol superstar Joe Dallesandro, with a real zipper attached to the album cover. You can see the bulge to the left of the zipper—but when you open the zipper up, there's only cardboard.

The best sight gag in Rob Reiner's rock & roll movie parody, *This Is Spinal Tap,* is a bulging-crotch gag. One of the band members gets stopped at the metal detector at the airport. He takes the metal objects out of his pockets and still he sets the system off. Finally an airport worker goes over him with a handheld detector, which beeps when it nears the bulge in his crotch. Reluctantly he reaches inside his pants and pulls out a large (presumably metal) cucumber.

PENIS CULTURE

GROUPIES

Rock & roll bands started traveling the country in the 1960s, playing cities large and small. Groupies followed them; they figured out ways to get backstage to meet the bands that played their hometowns, and tried to have sex with the band members. If no band member was available, even a member of the road crew would be a notch on a groupie's belt. Some groupies traveled with bands; some ended up marrying band members.

Being a groupie became an occupation of sorts in the 1960s. A young woman who was a groupie could be sexually active and aggressive and gain a certain kind of social approval for it because she was connecting herself with worldly power. The power was the rock star's cock.

One groupie, Cynthia Plaster Caster, had the wit to memorialize some of these power symbols in plaster, and the penis plaster cast became her art form. Her work is discussed in more detail in Chapter 4, "Penises in Art."

INDECENT EXPOSURE

At the same time that the '60s counterculture saluted the power of the penis, it also strove to get beyond such outmoded concepts as penis power, so that people could really get naked with each other, physically and emotionally. But really getting naked is a tall order at the best of times. Jan Hodenfield, who wrote about rock & roll for *Rolling Stone* and the *New York Post,* said to me, "Although no one talked about it as such, the idea was we were going to get down. And the secret of the dick would be peeled away. That's what John Lennon's album with Yoko, *Two Virgins,* was about. They were both naked on the cover— it was 'Here it is, here I am, I'm not hiding anything.' And nobody knew what to do about it."

A few months after *Two Virgins* was released, and undeterred by its reception, Jim Morrison of the Doors threatened to expose his cock to an audience of Miami teenagers. His biographers claim he was doing it to alter consciousness; besides, he only planned to strip down to his boxer shorts, and he only got as far as unbuckling his belt; in any case he was drunk. But his gesture was widely misunderstood. For various teens in his audience the wish became the deed, and they thought they'd actually seen him take out his cock and shake it at them. He was convicted of indecent exposure; he died of a drug overdose before he could be sentenced.

TIGHT JEANS

Tight jeans with a discernible cock, a perennially popular look with blue-collar workers and cowboys, has also remained a big gay fashion, since it makes cruising easier. "It used to be the style," a gay man told me, "that the cock would be hanging down one side or the other. Sometimes the jeans were strategically bleached to highlight it. Now it's the style that it's in the middle, because of the way the underwear is worn. It kind of creates a pouch, and it's the pouch and the size of the pouch, not the size of the outline of the dick, that's important." The Calvin Klein ad for Jockey shorts that covered a Times Square billboard in 1993, presenting a pouch with a cock and balls inside it several stories high, fixed this look forever in the memory of all who saw it. (The model was Mark Wahlberg.)

MALE VANITY

Part of being manly used to mean being unconcerned with one's appearance. Men still like to subscribe to that position, but ever since the 1960s the taboos against male vanity have been crumbling. Men don't care about appearance, and they also go to the gym and develop their bodies; they get expensive haircuts, facials and manicures; they spend money on clothes. In fact, by the late 1990s we were experiencing what the *New York Times* called a "Men's Fashion Boom." Men were becoming more concerned with fashion, just as women seemed to be getting sick of it. Between 1989 and 1996, the *Times* said in April 1997, while sales of women's clothing fell 10 percent, men's clothing sales increased by 21.3 percent.

In the November 1997 *Vogue*, Julie Baumgold, writing about male vanity, quoted anthropologist Lionel Tiger: "Once men could fairly well control their destiny through providing resources to women, but now that the female is obliged to create a living, he himself becomes a resource. He becomes his own product: Is he good-looking? Does he smell good? Before, when he had to provide for the female, he could have a potbelly. Now he has to appear attractive in the way the female had to be."

The more men care about appearance, the more their body parts become fair game.

Accompanying Baumgold's article was a series of photographs of the beautiful male movie star Brad Pitt. Pitt, she pointed out, has purposely taken roles that might neutralize his beauty, since that isn't all he wants to be known for.

Also in 1997 *Playgirl* published ten photographs of Brad Pitt. They were taken with a telephoto lens, and showed him romping naked on a Caribbean Island with his then-girlfriend Gwyneth Paltrow. Any fan who wanted could see Brad Pitt's penis. Pitt sued, claiming invasion of privacy and infliction of emotional distress, and a California court ordered *Playgirl* to recall the issue. Recall proved to be impossible, since the issue had long ago sold out on newsstands.

AMERICAN PENIS WORSHIP

This blossoming interest in the penises of movie stars, which in some people may border on the obsessive, seems to be the modern American version of communal penis worship. Considering, in addition, the amount of attention it's currently being paid, in art, literature and popular culture, you could say the penis itself has come into fashion.

PART

THREE

CUSTOMIZED

PENISES

W hen your sex organs stick out in front of you they may be easy to display, but they're also vulnerable. They just sit there, asking to be tampered with. And that's exactly what some men do—they take the part of themselves they love the best, the one by which they measure their manhood, and tamper with it.

Circumcision and castration are age-old male practices. Men go in for genital piercing and tattooing in a bigger way than women, and they also more often resort to transgender surgery. In researching this section I tried to find out why men would do such things. I also interviewed two transsexuals, about penis acquisition and penis disposal.

CHAPTER

EIGHT

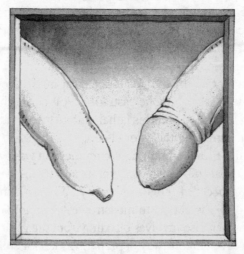

CIRCUMCISION AND CASTRATION

Circumcision is something men do to other men, and they do it to keep the male society functioning properly. Older men dominate younger men by hurting their penises; then they allow them to join the hurt-penis club.

I confess I had trouble at first getting close to the subject of circumcision. I had almost the same aversion to it that men have to menstruation—it seemed on the one hand inconsequential, on the other too dark, nasty and male. But obviously circumcision is important to men. At various times in their histories, circumcision was performed by Melanesians, Polynesians, Africans, natives of New Guinea —and possibly by native Americans in North and South America. Egyptians were practicing circumcision as early as the fifth century B.C., when the Greek mathematician

CUSTOMIZED PENISES

Pythagoras was circumcised before being allowed to study in the Egyptian temples. Currently Jews and Muslims practice circumcision, as do Coptic Christians and many tribal peoples. Most baby doctors in the U.S. routinely circumcise infants, unless somebody stops them.

Circumcision was a matter of great interest to Freud, who saw it as a symbolic castration. A nick on the penis warned the son to obey his father, and to give up all hopes of seducing his mother—or else.

Bruno Bettelheim thought circumcision was a way for men in tribal cultures to incorporate into themselves some envied aspects of female sexuality. Women can't have babies until they begin to menstruate—therefore circumcision, which also involves bleeding from the genitals, can be seen as a symbolic way of preparing men for childbirth.

Outside of the industrialized West, circumcision is almost always understood as an initiation rite; traditionally a boy who has been circumcised has become a member of his tribe. He and his dick, and the dicks of all his tribesmen, are now blood brothers. Men who are circumcised in a culture where most men are not, or who are uncircumcised in a culture where most men are, may feel like outsiders, and in fact may be perceived that way. In a number of tribes where circumcision is practiced, the children of the uncircumcised are considered to be illegitimate, or may even be abandoned or murdered at birth.

CIRCUMCISION BY FIRE

The Nandi of East Africa circumcise boys between the ages of fourteen and nineteen. The ritual, performed once every four and a half years, was described in 1939 by Felix Bryk in *Dark Rapture: The Sex-Life of the African Negro*. The night before the ceremony, everyone dances until they drop. Early in the morning the candidates bathe in the river, then dress in beads, brass plates and garlands of flowers. Then they're taken to the forest to the place where circumcisions are performed. Here they're grilled about their sexual experience. White clay and milk is rubbed into the head of each candidate, who kneels in front of a roaring fire. The circumciser's assistant pulls on the boy's foreskin, while the circumciser "grabs the glowing iron out of the fire and passes it around the foreskin until it falls off. The assistant throws it away while the master applies udder fat to the wound. During this operation, which is performed very rapidly, the candidate dares not cry out for if he did he would be mercilessly pierced through with a spear."

The initiates live in a hut together for six months while their wounds heal and they're tutored in the ways of men. After that, they're bound to each other for life.

THE CIRCUMCISING HERON

In Senegal, the Ehing people perform a circumcision ceremony, called Kombutsu, every twenty-five years. This ceremony and its meaning is described in *The Hatchet's Blood,* by Marc R. Schloss. "It is Kombutsu," Schloss says, "that determines the ritual rights of an elder and not chronological age, a point graphically illustrated by the plight of a man in another village who had missed the previous initiation and so had had, for all this time and in spite of his gray beard, the ritual status of a child."

On the day of Kombutsu, elders always say, a heron disguised as a person comes to meet the initiates. Amid much celebrating the initiates are taken one by one into the sacred part of the bush where, they are told, they're going to wrestle the heron. There are five or six "herons," and they use knives to cut the initiates' foreskins. Once an initiate has been cut, he's led to another part of the bush where his whole class sits on a termite hill; they're all fitted with splints made of twigs to make sure their penises don't heal crooked.

The Ehing think of Kombutsu as the male version of birth. Because Kombutsu dramatizes the male powers of generation, the cloths the men wear while their wounds are healing are said to make women fertile and prevent miscarriages.

SUBINCISION

Among the most radical of penis initiations is subincision, practiced by Australian Aborigines. In this rite, a man's urethra is slit open along the underside of his penis with a stone knife. The initial cut may be only an inch long, but eventually the urethra is opened from the head to the root of the penis; think of a butterflied hot dog. Often the men who've had the first, smallish cut are energized when they witness the next crop having the smallish cut, and demand to be cut down to the root this time. Most tribes that practice subincision consider the blood from the subincision opening to be the same as menstrual blood. "In New Guinea," Bruno Bettelheim says, "the penis is periodically incised, the operation usually being referred to as 'men's menstruation.' All avoidances imposed on women during the menstrual period also apply to men while they bleed from the incision wound." Like menstrual blood, blood from a subincision wound is considered to be powerfully connected to the source of life and may be used for healing purposes.

CIRCUMCISION AND CASTRATION

Men who have been subincised must squat when they urinate. In the days before men knew how to build fires, Bettelheim says, they had to be stopped from the pleasure of pissing on the fires they found, which would put them out and destroy their source of heat and light. A subincised man can't piss on a fire.

Subincision also changes the shape of a penis. Australian Aboriginal women are said to prefer having sex with partners who are subincised, presumably because penis width is greater—but subincision is not practiced in order to give the women pleasure.

One theory has it that Aborigines in Australia and New Guinea practice subincision to imitate their totem animal, the kangaroo, which has a two-headed dick. This theory is known as "kangaroo bifid penis envy."

OTHER PENIS MUTILATION CEREMONIES

The Dowayos, a people of the Cameroons, don't just circumcise their penises, they flay the whole shaft. When the men come back from this initiation, months later, they tell the women they had something done to their anuses. The women know what's actually happened, and joke about it. No one sees the flayed penises because from circumcision until the day they die the men wear penis sheaths, and they have intercourse in the dark. Like many peoples, the Dowayos believe civilization came to them when they started circumcising. Dowayo rainmaking and funeral ceremonies are based on the circumcision ceremony.

Each year at an initiation festival devoted to the hunting and killing of the dik-dik, the Ethiopian Konso

CUSTOMIZED PENISES

circumcise three grandfathers from priestly families. Only the tip of the foreskin is removed, but the ceremony, during which they wear skirts, changes the men's lives. When it's over they're no longer allowed to have sexual intercourse, and they're thought of as women. Some of them become transvestites. If the chosen men don't wish to participate in the ritual they can hire substitutes with similar qualifications. The Konso stratify their society so that a man's status, and that of his family, increases as he gets older. The custom of circumcising grandfathers may have originated as a way to prevent them from having children whose status would be too high at birth.

The Dogon of West Africa believe that the foreskin contains a man's female soul, and the clitoris a woman's maleness. They resolve the identity problems of both sexes with circumcision.

Some Polynesian societies, and the Kikuyu of East Africa, practice superincision, slitting the top of the foreskin without cutting anything off. Polynesians say they perform the operation to keep the penis clean and odor-free. When a superincised penis is flaccid the foreskin is likely to flap around.

And for a slight digression, here's a bit of testicle lore. Among the Janjero of Ethiopia, a man who's had both nipples and one testicle removed may never rule. All males with the exception of the king and his sons are mutilated in this manner. Members of the lowest class are left alone, since no one would let them rule in any case.

JEWS

Jews perform circumcision on the eighth day after a boy child is born. They do so as a symbol of their covenant with God. In Genesis 17: 10–12, God says to Abraham, "This is my covenant, which you shall keep, between me and you and your descendants after you: Every male among you shall be circumcised. You shall be circumcised in the flesh of your foreskins, and it shall be a sign of the covenant between me and you. He that is eight days old among you shall be circumcised. . . ."

Jewish infants have their foreskins cut off in a ceremony called a *bris*. The rite is performed by a *mohel*, and the family invites friends. For the first two thousand years of Jewish circumcision only the tip of the foreskin was removed. Michelangelo's *David,* who seems uncircumcised, looks the way circumcised Jews used to look. In fact, it was so easy for Jewish boys to stretch their foreskins out and pass as uncircumcised that finally, around 140 A.D., the rabbis changed the law. At that point *mohels* began taking off the entire foreskin. This practice made it clear who was a Jew and who wasn't—and during World War II Jewish men, trying to escape the Nazis, suffered for it.

MUSLIMS

The prophet Mohammed was circumcised, and although Islam does not demand circumcision, it is considered a sign of purity and is faithfully practiced. Most converts to Islam are circumcised as a first step. Thirteen used to be the proper age for circumcising a Muslim boy, because Ishmael, the father of the Arab peoples, was thirteen when he was circumcised by his father, Abraham.

In Turkey during the seventeenth century, Christian residents had to pay a tax. To decide who was taxable, tax collectors often stopped strangers and asked them to show their circumcision.

CUSTOMIZED PENISES

A few years ago I was in Istanbul in August, and every once in a while we would see a family in an open car with a boy resplendently dressed, and I'd be told he was going to his circumcision. Turkish circumcisions take place during the summer, while school is out. Sometimes groups are circumcised together. A rich family might hire a hall for the event. Boys are dressed in capes and carry scepters and wear hats inscribed with the prayer "Massalah" (Allah preserve him). The morning of the ceremony a boy is taken through town on horseback or in a car, followed if possible by musicians. He goes back home to be circumcised by a surgeon, and when it's done he's kept amused by friends and family and given presents. Guests are feasted following the circumcision. Festivities last several days, until the boy is recovered.

Sir Richard Burton, the nineteenth-century British Orientalist, described the Islamic circumcision ritual performed in Sind in the Indus Valley. An eight-year-old boy, "dressed in saffron-coloured clothes and adorned with Sihra [a paper or flower garland], is mounted on horseback, and led round the town to the sound of instruments, singing and firing of guns. When he returns home the barber performs the operation in the same way as done in India, but not nearly so skillful [sic]. Clarified butter, wax and the leaves of the Neem tree are used as dressing to the wound, which is expected to heal in eight or ten days."

USES OF THE FORESKIN

Says Sir Richard Burton's biographer Edward Rice, "Burton noted that the Pathans buried the foreskin in a damp part of the house where the water jars were kept, possibly in the hope that it would grow and add to the boy's virility. In other areas of the Punjab it was tossed on the roof of the house or tied to it by a straw. The Muslims of Delhi tied the foreskin to the boy's left foot with a peacock feather so that no evil shadow would fall on him. The Brahuis, a Dravidian people of the north who attracted Burton's interest, either buried the foreskin under a tree so that the boy would be fruitful in generation or in damp earth to cool the burning pain of the wound."

During the Middle Ages the foreskin of Jesus Christ was said to reside at the Abbey Church of Coulombs, in Chartres. According to legend this holy foreskin made a woman fruitful, and also gave her an easy delivery. Henry V of Agincourt borrowed the foreskin when his wife, Catherine of France, was about to give birth, in order to ease her labor. Things went so well with Catherine that when Henry returned the relic he had a sanctuary built for its repose.

After circumcision the Poro people of Liberia dry the foreskins, which are then cooked and eaten by the girls of the tribe as part of their initiation. Likewise, the clitoris and labia minora removed from the girls during initiation are dried, cooked and eaten by the boys at circumcision. "As is often the case in oral incorporation," Bruno Bettelheim says, "it is difficult to decide which desire is stronger, the hostile desire to take away from the other sex, or the envious desire to possess the incorporated parts."

In the U.S. in the 1990s biomedical companies use infant foreskins in the manufacture of insulin. Cells from infant foreskins are also used to grow artificial skin for burn patients. One foreskin supplies enough genetic material for 250,000 square feet of skin.

TO CIRCUMCISE
OR NOT

Infant boys are regularly circumcised in hospitals in the United States because we believe the surgery promotes good health. A circumcised penis is easier to keep clean, and is thought to be less likely to contract venereal diseases and urinary tract infections. Circumcision also prevents the development of phimosis—a foreskin so tight it can't retract properly, making erection painful if not impossible and the discharge of semen difficult. (Louis XVI suffered from phimosis, which is why he and Marie Antoinette had no royal offspring until after 1778. By that time, according to the memoirs of Marie Antoinette's hairdresser, Louis had made an appointment to get circumcised, changed his mind and found a way to stretch his foreskin by himself.)

As recently as 1970 circumcision was still a mark of membership in the middle class, and 90 percent of American baby boys were circumcised. But research conducted in the past twenty years seems to indicate that circumcision may make no difference to a man's health. And the surgery has its drawbacks—it hurts, it's done to infants without anesthetic (as well as without their consent), and too often it's botched, sometimes in major ways. By 1992 the circumcision rate in the U.S. had dropped to 59 percent. It had become politically correct to leave your boy as nature intended him, and a vociferous anticircumcision movement was in place. This movement has two wings—parents and practitioners who don't want to hurt infants unnecessarily; and angry circumcised men who want their foreskins back.

FORESKINS AND SEX

Having a foreskin probably increases the intensity of sexual pleasure, though not necessarily its duration. The glans, covered by a foreskin, is more sensitive to touch, and the sensation of the foreskin sliding against the glans is said to be deeply thrilling.

As previously noted, foreskins are an important part of sex for some gay men—and a magazine called *Foreskin Quarterly* caters to these men. In it, men with foreskins stretch them out with their hands. They hold the foreskin out invitingly, a pale, translucent funnel of skin. One practice in gay sex is for one man to pull his foreskin over the head of the other man's dick. This is called docking. A foreskin can also easily be pierced and ringed for use in sadomasochistic practices.

Foreskins don't matter that much to most women, who, when it comes to penises, can get used to almost anything. But three of the women I talked with had strong opinions. One thought all men should be uncut. "As far as feeling goes it's not a lot different except there's less friction when it goes for a long time," she said. "But psychologically it makes a huge difference to know it's untouched, undamaged socially, unfettered."

The second disagreed. "Uncircumcised dicks are harder to go down on," she said. "Because they have folds. And you don't know what you're going to find there."

So did the third: "It's so much more hygienic circumcised. And the penis is so much more accessible. Otherwise you have to wash it all the time, and you can't have as much spontaneous sex. Also I like to nibble and bite on the head of a man's penis, as if it was an ice-cream cone.

I like to actually chew on it. If a man cannot be bit on his penis because there's a foreskin in the way I would feel deprived of something."

UNCIRCUMCISING

In the olden days men were either circumcised or they weren't, and it never occurred to them they had a choice about it. But now we have options for everything—and one option available to men who hate being circumcised, or feel they were victimized as infants when some doctor strapped them down and cut their foreskins off, is foreskin restoration. A man can have plastic surgery to restore his foreskin. Or he can do it himself, following instructions in *The Joy of Uncircumcising*, by Jim Bigelow, Ph.D. There are several good foreskin restoration web sites he can visit, if he needs moral support.

Bigelow, a clinical psychologist who restored his own foreskin, believes the process can be vital to a man's mental health. "The penis is often involved in the negative self-image of males who feel in some way bad about themselves," he says. For men who "grew up wondering what was so wrong with them or their penis that something had to be cut off of them," foreskin restoration can also provide "a sense of regained power. That little baby boy is not strapped to that board or being held down anymore. He's . . . getting back as much as can possibly be regained of what they took from him. He's in charge now!"

To bring his foreskin back, according to Bigelow, a man essentially has to keep pulling on what's left of it. The recommended method is to stretch whatever remains of the foreskin over the head and tape it down. After it's lengthened to a certain point, weights and foam rubber cones may also be used.

A complete recovery might take as little as four months or as much as four years, most likely later rather than sooner. And a taped-down dick imposes certain limitations. In fact, the entire restoration period resembles a penis ritual of grand proportions. When the man wants to have sex he must pull the tape off, and if this irritates his skin too much he can only have sex when the tape comes off by itself. To urinate he can either sit down, or dribble. Boxer shorts are the preferred underwear to accommodate the program. Men who insist on Jockeys, and are using weights, must cut a hole in the Jockey pouch and let the dick with its weight hang on the outside.

And then, once the process is complete, the new foreskin rarely hugs the glans the way nature intended, and needs to be replaced by hand. To correct this condition a man can have a surgical touch-up. Some men pull the groin skin so far down the shaft that they end up with pubic hair on their dicks and need electrolysis.

But according to Bigelow the results are worth it. "My men report that from the very first time they applied the tape, their glans felt warm and sheltered, as nature intended. . . . They say that they cannot imagine having their glans exposed again and not enjoying that 'at home' feeling they've discovered."

Bigelow's book is full of testimonials from men— young, old, heterosexual, homosexual—who've successfully restored their foreskins.

And yet the results of a study published in the *Journal of the American Medical Association* in 1997 make it seem that circumcised men have more fun. Even after religion and social class were factored in, they reportedly engaged in a wider range of sexual practices, like oral and anal sex and masturbation. They were also less likely to lose interest in sex as they got older. Dr. Edward O. Laumann, who conducted the study at the University of Chicago, told the *New York Times* there were two possible explanations for the variations. Either uncircumcised men, still a minority in the U.S., felt stigmatized and therefore inhibited, or circumcised men had to be more inventive to make up for the reduced sensitivity in their dicks.

CASTRATION

'Twas Christmas in the harem and the eunuchs all were
    there
Sitting on the stairway looking at the maidens fair.
The sultan entered the harem and he shouted through the
    halls,
What do you want for Christmas? And the eunuchs
    shouted, Balls!

In many ancient cultures when you won a battle and killed a man you cut off his dick as a trophy. There are friezes more than three thousand years old on the walls of the smaller temple across the way from Karnak, in Egypt, showing piles of enemy penises. Accompanying the penises are hands, which those enemies may have used to pleasure themselves. At the end of the nineteenth century, Peter C. Remondino wrote in his *History of Circumcision, From the Earliest Times to the Present,* "Among the modern Berbers it is still a practice for a young man, on proposing marriage, to exhibit to his prospective father-in-law the virile members of all the enemies he has overcome, as evidence of his manhood and right to the title of warrior." In one Ethiopian culture, as recently as 1972, the penises of vanquished enemies were worn by the victor on a bracelet.

The cock and balls, everyone understood, was the seat of the enemy's manhood, and it was manhood that caused all the fighting.

There were even sects who practiced self-castration. The Skopsy, a Russian Christian group of the nineteenth century, cut off their own genitals to show the strength of their dedication to God.

In ancient Rome, novitiate priests of the goddess Cybele castrated themselves with swords to the accompaniment of music and chanting. In medieval Syria, young Christian men sliced off their own genitals during religious orgies, then ran through the streets with their organs in their hands until they selected a house to fling them into. As if it weren't enough having a bloody severed dick land on your doorstep, the people of the chosen house were then expected to take the new eunuch in and dress him as a woman.

Castration—either by simply removing the balls or by taking off the penis as well—was also practiced as an early form of bioengineering. Men without sex organs, it was found, were more governable and also had better powers of concentration. The blood couldn't rush to their dicks if they had no dicks, and even if they did have dicks, without their balls there was no testosterone to drive them crazy with lust. There were four ways of creating eunuchs: complete shaving of penis and testicles (these men had to use quills to urinate); removal of the balls alone; severing of the penis alone; crushing of the testicles (this had to be done when a boy was young). The operations were dangerous, particularly if the penis was removed, and many died from them.

CUSTOMIZED PENISES

Eunuchs were almost always people in subordinate positions—either conquered people taken as slaves, or boys who were surgically altered in order to serve their rulers. Being castrated in the latter case was a way up the social ladder—you traded your sexuality for a species of refinement. You became a not-man, an unthreatening man and therefore theoretically more useful.

A man whose balls were removed before puberty would not be likely to develop an adult penis. He would also retain his pure, strong, boyish soprano. Boys with singing talent were castrated in eighteenth- and nineteenth-century Italy in the hope they would end up singing in the Papal Choir or the opera. Those who became opera stars were idolized—and besieged by admirers, male and female, who found their sexual strangeness mesmerizing. They also apparently had love affairs. At least they did in the movie *Farinelli* and in the Anne Rice novel *Cry to Heaven*. (In *Farinelli* the castrato even sort-of fathers a child, doing his own lovemaking, then calling in his brother to deposit the semen. Anne Rice's castrati have sex with each other, with men who have balls and with women. Their penises are described as shorter than average, but thick.)

Eunuchs worked as civil servants for the Chinese emperors, and were appointed by Byzantine emperors as government ministers and even Church patriarchs. In most places where rulers had harems, eunuchs guarded the harems. Though eunuchs could not impregnate women, those who still had penises might well be capable of sexual arousal and prolonged lovemaking. A sultan might have hundreds of concubines. Unless she was a favorite, a woman in his employ had a chance of having sex with him maybe twice a year. And so some of them had passionate love affairs with eunuchs, the only other men they were allowed to see.

Chinese eunuchs, who were totally shaved, kept their privates preserved inside sealed jars, and when they died the jars were buried with them. They might also be required to show the contents of their jars—which they referred to as "the precious"—as qualifications for job promotion.

Eunuchs could get work with various absolute monarchs until the early twentieth century, when, with the death of the Chinese and Ottoman Empires, their market dried up.

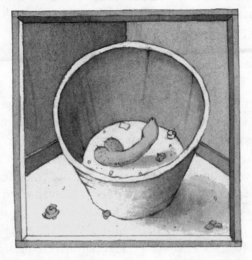

MALE-TO-
FEMALE: AN
INTERVIEW
WITH BABY
DEE

Baby Dee worked as a church organist when she was a man, running the choirs and teaching music to children. Now, thanks to surgical intervention, she's a woman, and a lot more outgoing. She's in her middle forties, tall and broad-shouldered, with a handsome face, shoulder-length blond hair and beautiful skin, and she makes a living as a street entertainer. Summer nights she can be seen pedaling around Greenwich Village and SoHo on an over-size tricycle with a concert harp hung on the back; when she stops she plays the accordion and sings.

I wanted her perspective on the differences between having a penis and not having one.

Q: When you were a man were you straight or gay?

A: I wasn't gay, that's for certain. I would sometimes be in a situation where a gay man would come on to me, and it would make me feel like a girl, so I would like that, but it would never work because it's not true, he didn't like me because I'm a girl, he liked me because I'm a guy. So that would be a terrible disappointment.

Q: Did you have sexual relationships with women?

A: Basically the women I would involve myself with were women I wanted to be rather than women I wanted to be with. That's not a healthy premise for a relationship. As a matter of fact it's not a relationship—not in any direct way. In terms of the body, I hated my body. I hated it. I hated having a dick.

Q: Why?

A: Well . . . it's not very ladylike. Obviously for most men it's the source of their joy. For me it was absolutely the opposite. Having a penis was just frustrating in every way. If I would feel any kind of sexual arousal, obviously I'd get a hard-on. Which I would hate. So nothing made any sense. I could have sex with women but I'd have to have a fantasy of being the woman to do it. I tried to eke out a life as a guy. I didn't do anything about it until I was thirty-six, thirty-seven, and I started to see a shrink and it all came out.

Q: When did you have the surgery?

A: About two years ago, after a transition period of taking female hormones. When you have the surgery they remove your testicles. Everything else is basically inverted.

Q: And they throw out the testicles?

A: Yeah. In the shit can. I didn't have any problem with that whatsoever. When your gender and your body hook up and are the same it's a good thing. You inhabit your body. That's the way I am now. Now I can't imagine myself having a penis. Because I never inhabited it when I had it. Mentally it was never there. At the same time I don't consider myself to be a regular girl or however you want to describe it. I'm obviously not like other women. But I'll be goddamned if I'll be lumped in with men. No matter what I am, I *am* female.

Q: Do you have a sex life with men now?

A: Sometimes. The better part of a year after I had my surgery it was like a field trip. I went hog wild. For a while I was into the S&M scene, and what I noticed was, all these dominant guys, guys who basically like to beat up on women in socially acceptable ways, all have these tiny dicks. There wasn't one who didn't. Isn't that amazing?

Actually for a transsexual, in terms of having relationships, you're much better off having a dick, because then at least you have a value on the sex market. There are men, a lot of them, who are very turned on by the idea of a woman with a dick. Men in the company of other men will avoid such creatures, but if you did it on a one-on-one basis, probably ninety percent of men would be interested enough to act on it.

Q: They say men are led around by their dicks. Were you? How did that feel?

A: It's like being tied to a St. Bernard. It's like having a pit bull on a leash that's attached to your body, which you have to walk every day, and I'm very happy not to have a penis. I mean, now that I don't have one I love penises, but I just like them on other people, not me. I really feel sorry for the guys who have them. Because what are they

121

for? They're for women. Physically for a guy sex is about getting rid of something. Something leaves the guy. I always felt that woman is really at the center of the thing. Guys are like outsiders.

Q: *But they're sexually dominant. When a man is sexually excited it's very hard to stop him beyond a certain point.*

A: I kind of like that about men. It's beautiful in its animal sense, that men are driven to do this thing in a way that goes against their thoughts or feelings or whatever. The sexiest men I've known have an animal quality. But very few men are comfortable with that real animal quality. I love to be overpowered by a man, and to be under the will of this guy, but usually it's just some scrawny little jerk with a bad attitude. Whereas there are men out there who are really powerful in their body and totally connect with it and can dominate with total goodwill. All men should be like that, and maybe under all their neuroses they are all like that.

Q: *Now that you're a woman can you have orgasms?*

A: Oh, yeah. It's just as earthshaking, it's just as big a deal. It's not a subtle thing, it's huge. It's more all over and it's more deep inside, and for me it's more satisfying. But that may just be me, since I didn't like being a guy.

Q: *All the symbols of power in the world are in the shape of a phallus. Isn't it hard to give up that worldly power?*

A: I think I still have a lot of that power. For instance, the act that I do on my tricycle—very few genetic women could get away with that. The thing about men is, men take up a huge amount of space. I'm five-eleven, and there is a lot of maleness built into me. You know, that over-the-top drag queen thing—it may be a parody of women, but it's also just a male version. It's taking a woman and incorporating that pushy, space-taking-up maleness into it. I guess in a way that is partaking of the power that men have, even though I don't have a dick.

Q: But you have a different point of view from most people.

A: One of the things you learn when you go through the transsexual process is the way people are ruled by their gender—and it's a fiercely tyrannical thing. Men have to fit in with men as men, and women have to fit in with women as women. "Normal" people spend a lot of time studying how to do that. It's very hard for a man to just see a woman he likes and go after her; it doesn't really work that way. Men gauge what they want by what other men want and they line up their desire with other men, because their real desire is to fit in with other men, more than to fuck the girls. People find that hard to believe but it's true. And the same with women. Women think of themselves as being ruled by men and men think of themselves as being ruled by women, but it's not that way at all. Everybody is imprisoned in their gender, and they haven't got a clue. Either you're in it or you're going against it, but clarity along those lines does not come cheap.

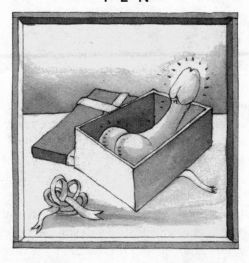

FEMALE-TO-MALE: AN INTERVIEW WITH "JACK"

When I interviewed "Jack" he was twenty-six, and had been taking testosterone for two years. He had male facial hair and a young man's voice and manner, and was living as a man while he looked forward to body-modifying surgery. He was also becoming reconciled to the fact that the one thing he wanted most, a real penis, would never be his. I asked him first about the steps of the transformation from female to male:

CUSTOMIZED PENISES

A: You start by taking testosterone, and you're usually on hormones for a year or two. Then you have a bilateral mastectomy and they reconstruct the chest so you look like a man. The next step is usually a hysterectomy, and after that, once you're not producing estrogen, you can lower the testosterone dosage. Then you can have a metoidioplasty. They remove the hood of the clitoris, which has become enlarged from the testosterone so it's maybe the length of the thumb, two inches; but only about an inch of it sticks out of the body. When they remove the hood the whole two inches extends from the body. Also with the metoidioplasty a lot of guys get saline testicular implants. Most of a man's heft comes from the balls, not the dick, so if you have balls you feel a presence there. With the testicular implants they close up the vagina and remove the cervix. They construct the testicles with the outer labia. The enlarged clitoris acts like a very small penis basically; it becomes erect.

Q: *Do you ejaculate?*

A: No. Without a penis it doesn't work that way. You can't really penetrate anybody. It's a two-inch dick. But it's as sensitive as a clitoris and probably more so because there's more of it and also the testosterone really increases the sex drive and the sexual response. I went to a girls' Catholic high school and I went to Mount Holyoke. I got a feminist education and I didn't really want to believe men think differently from women. But especially when I first started with the hormones, I couldn't stop thinking about sex, it was just constant. I was like a fifteen-year-old boy. Before, I used to see women on the subway and I would have a thought process—she's attractive, I would like to get to know her—and it would be sort of narrative. With the testosterone the narrative is gone—it's just flashes of these sexual, aggressive images. Just bang-bang-bang in your head. For the first six months or so I found myself leering at women. I used to think, You don't have to leer, couldn't you be less obvious about it? But you just want to look. And you find that orgasms come a lot quicker. It used to take half an hour, warming up. But now ten minutes is all I need. Men get criticized for coming too fast, but I think it's hormonal.

Q: You look like a man. You use the men's room, right?

A: I use the men's room, and if I went into a women's room they would scream at me and kick me out. But I don't have a penis. I cannot use a men's room if it doesn't have a stall. For me, peeing is going to be a lifelong problem. I go to a female-to-male therapy group, and we've devoted hours to peeing. You find out that many men pee sitting down, every time. So you think, Well, that's okay. But even so, when I started using men's rooms I felt really nervous, like I was going to be found out, that my pee would somehow sound different hitting the water. And we talked about it in group, and we realized that women pay attention to each other in the women's bathroom, but men don't pay attention to anybody in the men's bathroom. When they're standing up peeing at the urinal, they burp and they fart, they whistle, they talk to themselves. A gay man's pickup bathroom is a different situation, but you go into the men's room at Yankee Stadium, and they're going in, they're peeing, they're getting out. They're not talking to anybody, they're not making eye contact with anybody, they don't say hello. They hardly stop to wash their hands.

Q: Is your roommate transsexual also?

A: No, he's genetic. I worked with him at my first job out of grad school. I transitioned on the job. Then, when I switched to my new job, a year ago, I interviewed as a man and that's all they know. As a man I get treated differently. I used to be expected to be good at filing, and typing, and answering the phone. Now, if I'm well organized, and good at answering the telephone, they think it's fabulous. I am expected to be more aggressive, I'm expected to speak up at meetings, which I don't know how to do. It's funny—I have the power that goes with having a penis, but I haven't got one. Just walking through life with my clothes on I'm a straight white male, and what nobody knows is that I belong to just about the smallest sexual minority, simultaneously.

Q: As a straight white male, are there other things you do that you couldn't do before?

A: One thing I do is go to topless bars with my male friends. And I can see that men looking at the female body in many ways feel very powerless before it. I think that men looking at women are looking at a mystery. Because men in topless bars, unless they're in a pack and they're drinking, are not at all rowdy, the way you would think. It's almost as if they're in a church. They don't say a word, they just look. In awe. It's really almost beautiful. Men want to look at naked women. Women have the power to be naked before men and render them silent up on that stage.

I think, having gone through that first onslaught of testosterone, that men are really afraid of their sexuality. Because those first feelings are so overwhelming and strong you feel like a monster, you feel like you could rape a woman. You walk down the street and you're looking at women in short dresses and you just feel like you're going to explode, you have to repress it constantly. And it goes away but there's always this longing for a woman, it's constant, this hunter thing.

Q: I guess a hard-on is the physical expression of that longing.

A: I do have them, but to a lesser degree—I have an inch and a half. Female-to-males also experience what's called the phantom penis. You feel as if you have one, it's so real. When you're very sexually excited you feel as if it's really there. And then you reach down, and it's not there. You dream about it. I have dreams about having a penis, and in the dreams it's funny-looking, it's particularly long or particularly narrow or it's curled and it's strange. In your dreams you have a penis, I guess the way someone without legs would dream about having legs. I know guys who pack regularly—they stuff their pants. They either stuff with a sock or they'll wear an actual dildo. I've tried that, but the act of trying to re-place what is not there only makes you think about it not being there.

Q: *Can't they make you a fake penis?*

A: You mean a phalloplasty. It's about a hundred thousand dollars; insurance pays for none of that, and it doesn't really work. They construct it from skin from the lower abdomen, or the upper arm. They make it extra-long because it doesn't become erect, and so in order to have, say, a six-inch erect penis you have to have a six-inch flaccid penis. Then they'll add on a few inches to that because in many cases the end will turn black and need to be removed. It can't become erect, so what you do is you have a rod. I don't know, do you keep it under your pillow or something? When you want to have sex you insert the rod into the penis, I'm not sure how. In-stead of having a rod you can have a little pump they put into your hip or balls and you inflate and deflate an im-plant. I think the implant is more expensive than the rod. But the rod can come out. While you're having sex with a woman the rod can come right out, and then you have to get it out of her and put it back inside you. Making a

CUSTOMIZED PENISES

urethra involves very expensive microsurgery. So there's a lot of complications. But if you don't have one you still have to sit down to pee. And let's say your dick doesn't turn black and fall off, and let's say your urethra doesn't close up, and let's say you go home and nothing goes wrong. You've got something that looks like a really ugly dick, like an Italian sausage, or something Lorena Bobbitt got to but didn't finish off, and you may or may not be able to feel anything with it. The guys I know who've had it done don't seem to have much more luck with girlfriends than the guys who haven't.

Q: How do you have sex?

A: Well, I don't very much, yet. That's still a problem. When I lived as a lesbian, in high school and college, I always had girlfriends. Now I'm just coming out of my awkward second adolescence. For a while I looked like a teenager, kind of gawky, and nobody really looked at me. Now I notice people are interested in me; older gay men really check me out, so I know I look all right. In the two years I've been transitioning I dated one woman briefly, and I guess you would say we had sex like lesbians do. I'm not comfortable with that definition of it, but basically the genitals are the same. A lot of guys don't allow their genitals to be touched at all when they're having sex. They use a strap-on dildo and have orgasms just from the friction of that rubbing against the clitoris.

Q: Why?

A: It just freaks you out. You hate them, you don't want them. Those feelings come up for me, too, but physically it feels good, so I'm going to use what I have. But before I started transitioning I was basically impotent for a couple of years. I had a girlfriend who would have been happy to have sex, but I was repulsed by her body because it looked

130

like mine. And my body was keeping me from being who I wanted to be. You feel like your body's betraying you. When I was thirteen and I got my period I just felt so ashamed. My body was doing things I didn't want it to do. The testosterone, thank God, stops my period. So that's good. The money I spend on hormones I save on tampons.

CHAPTER
ELEVEN

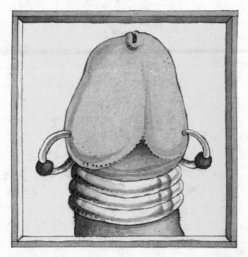

DESIGN YOUR
OWN DICK

"I think it's impossible for human beings to progress un-less there are certain magical events that occur periodi-cally. . . . Those events are called rites of passage—initiation. . . . Some people instinctively know this, and if society won't give them a rite of passage, they'll invent one! It must be physical, it must be painful, it must be bloody, and it should leave a mark. Those are characteristics of a rite of passage."

—*Fakir Musafar, quoted in* Modern Primitives

PENIS PIERCING

Western men have their penises pierced for many reasons, and one reason is the way it looks. There are men who, when they dress up, can put silver studs in rows up and down their penis shafts, studs in the glans, rings through the urethra, rings all over the balls. You can see photographs of these men and their hardware in certain issues of *PFIQ* (*Piercing Fans International Quarterly*), published by the venerable Gauntlet piercing parlors.

Many men with pierced penises also like the way it feels to have sex, or just to sit around, with a piece of jewelry inserted into their private parts. As Brian Murphy, master piercer and store manager of Gauntlet in New York, explained it to me, "You're creating a tube of tissue where there was no sensation before. You're going to get pressure and tugging in areas where there was nothing. So you're increasing sensation, and creating a new and different feeling on top of the old one."

There are even some men who like the way it feels just being at the piercer and thinking about being pierced. In a 1978 interview in *PFIQ* the famous piercing and tattoo artist Mr. Sebastian said, "I realize quite a lot of people that come to be pierced find the actual piercing erotic. . . . One occasionally even encounters a very erect cock waiting to be pierced. I've had some that I've had to have jack off before the piercing. I would hesitate to do an ampallang or a Prince Albert [piercing techniques] on an erect cock because there would be so much extra blood up there."

Brian Murphy told me he sometimes encountered men who ejaculated while being prepped for piercing. "Usually it's out of their control," he said. "They're so worked up about getting the piercing it's just a function of their body. But some of them will get off before they're pierced and then they'll want their money back. And I say, 'I'm sorry.'"

Murphy sat in his small office facing lower Fifth Avenue. His arms were covered with handsome black tattoos. He had rings embedded in his earlobes, each lobe with a ring-finger-size hole in it, rimmed in gold. His soul patch, a small tuft of hair between lower lip and chin, stuck straight out. He looked smart, tasteful and efficient.

Penis piercings started in the gay community, he said, but now the customers are about half gay, half straight— and also half young, half older. About 10 or 15 percent of the burgeoning piercing business, he said, is genital. The rest is mainly nipples, and the navels, nostrils and tongues so popular with suburban teenagers.

Some penis piercing is done with forceps to hold the tissue in place, some is freehand. "For a frenum—where you pierce the skin on the underside of the penis—or for a scrotum piercing, you mark your dots and then you put forceps on and line the dots up in the forceps and then do the piercing into a cork. With a freehand piercing, after you mark the dots you don't use any tools except a needle —and your fingers. You line it up and do the piercing, pushing toward your fingers. Only a very experienced piercer should do a freehand piercing because the piercer is at a lot of risk, even though he's wearing latex gloves."

A penis piercing can take as little as four weeks or as much as six months to heal. During the healing period a latex barrier must be used for any sexual contact, even oral.

All customers for penis piercing want to know if it hurts, and the answer is yes, but it only hurts for a little while. Murphy said he never uses anesthetic, since it can distort the tissue, making the work come out crooked.

CUSTOMIZED PENISES

To look at a pierced penis you might think it had been injured or damaged, but the men who have them seem to think of these wounds as battle scars. The experience they went through in having the piercing proves they can take it. On the Internet, at sites devoted to body piercing, men describe their initiations, often conducted in the presence of their girlfriends or wives. They scream in pain and then come out the other side, renewed.

One man who posted an account of his experience on the Internet described getting an apadravya, which goes in under the corona and out the head: ". . . my penis felt like it was being ripped from the inside out—almost. . . . The piercing most likely only took 2–3 seconds but felt like 5–10 seconds! . . . And then, all of a sudden, I got this warm feeling—the endorphin rush."

Another man, who also got an apadravya, because his wife's genital piercing was a turn-on for them both, described the aftermath: ". . . peeing was essentially pain-less, though I did bleed a bit afterward, entirely through the top hole. . . . I've had my first hard-on, which was plea-surable. . . . My foreskin and glans seem to be much more sensitive—in a good way. . . . Attitude-wise, I'm far less self-conscious of my body. When nude, I feel more at ease, as if I were dressed."

THE AESTHETIC PENIS

There are men whose sexuality becomes dependent on penis jewelry. Murphy, who'd just moved to New York when I interviewed him, described his genitally bejeweled former customers in San Francisco. Usually they were older men, he said, who'd started when they were younger. "Some of these men have tons of jewelry and function fine without it. For others it's a question of what's going to turn you on more mentally—penetrating a partner or wearing all this jewelry. They might have found their kink is so extreme that it's the only way they can get off. So they don't have to worry about getting hard or staying hard or whether they're going to hurt somebody."

Penis jewelry can succeed in making a flaccid penis interesting. A penis decorated with rows of studs and rings looks more like an art object than a sex object. It becomes a kind of ceremonial weapon, or a thing encased in armor, which may express its owner's feeling about it.

THE ASCETIC PENIS

Modern Primitives, published in 1989 by Re/Search Publications, is devoted to body modification pioneers, none of whom is more assiduous in the pursuit of new sensations and their spiritual ramifications than Fakir Musafar. Fakir has worn a corset that reduced his waist to nineteen inches, he's hung by hooks through the piercings in his chest, he's lain on a bed of blades—all in the pursuit of altered states of consciousness.

According to Fakir, the sadhus—those Indians who elongate their penises with weights—hardly mind forgoing intercourse, since their stretched-out cocks keep them "aroused and on the verge of orgasm all the time, every day."

In his *Modern Primitives* interview, Fakir describes other practices that take a man beyond orgasm. One is "containment," when a sadhu rolls his scrotum in such a way that he can push his penis back inside his abdomen. Another, also performed in India, is "encasement," when a man seals his penis and testicles up in a brass ball with a small hole for urination. He can leave the ball on for months, and during all that time he'll be building up his primal energy because he won't be able to have an erection or an orgasm. Fakir says he once encased his genitals in plaster for just two days, and when he took off the encasement the slightest touch felt "incredible."

Another kind of body modification that's described as a sexual turn-on in *Modern Primitives* is ball-stretching. You use a steel ring weight at the top of the testicles. "Once it's on it feels like having your balls licked and sucked and being played with by someone's hand," according to Genesis P-Orridge, a cult figure on the industrial music scene and the leader of the band Throbbing Gristle. "You tend to have a semi hard-on all the time when you wear them." P-Orridge says he's seen photographs of a man wearing fourteen ring weights, and his testicles hang to his knees.

Also in *Modern Primitives* is a photograph of the genitals of a man who split his penis in half, giving it two heads. The man calls his modification "erotically exhilarating." He says he still has full erections, orgasms and ejaculations, but in two separate halves. "Entry into the vagina requires a little extra effort for insertion, but once my penis is inside, its opened effect on the vagina's inner lining is more pronounced, giving better female orgasmic feelings."

BASIC MALE GENITAL PIERCINGS

AMPALLANG—horizontal piercing through the center of the head, above the urethra and the erectile tissue.

APADRAVYA—vertical piercing through the penis head.

These piercings are common in Borneo, where the inserted pins may be made of bone or precious metals. In the West the pin is usually a metal rod with balls on either end. Ampallangs and apadravyas are said to increase sexual pleasure for women—but may cause difficulties with anal penetration.

DYDOE—piercing and studs through the corona (the rim around the head of the penis). Returns some of the sensitivity lost with circumcision; probably developed by Jewish medical students before World War II. This piercing is considered the most painful, and healing time is two to six months. Most men have it done on both sides of the head.

FRENUM—piercing through the loose piece of flesh on the underside of the penis behind the head, sometimes worn with barbells, or a ring that encircles the shaft just below the glans.

FORESKIN—piercing through the tip. With a ring through his foreskin a man can be pulled around by the dick. It moves to the top or side when the penis is erect.

PRINCE ALBERT—piercing through the urethra at the base of the glans on the underside. Jewelry, usually a ring or an L-bar (a half ring with balls at each end), goes through the base of the head and out the urethra. Called a "dressing ring" in Victorian times, it was used, with a piece of ribbon, to secure a man's penis to his leg and prevent an unsightly bulge under tight pants. Supposedly Prince Albert wore one, to pull his foreskin back from his glans and make hygiene easy. The most popular of penis piercings, it heals fast—in a month or two. May cause spraying during urination.

CUSTOMIZED PENISES

A penis cannot be pierced through the shaft without destroying the erectile tissue. Some men have the skin of the shaft pierced, and wear rings or studs in it. Some men also have the skin of their balls pierced and ringed.

PENIS INSERTS

SOUTHEAST ASIAN PENISES

The practice of inserting objects into the penis has a long history in Southeast Asia.

From the fourteenth to the seventeenth centuries, men around Burma and Thailand used to have metal bells, some as big as chicken eggs, put under the skin of their dicks. A man might wear as many as a dozen at a time; it was a great honor to receive, from the king, a bell he had worn in his penis and then removed for you.

In Sumatra, during the nineteenth and early twentieth centuries, men wore small objects under their penis skin, shaped like truncated pyramids and made of shell, stone or precious metals. In Sulawesi, another Indonesian Island, the Toraja wore rows of balls under the skin.

Men in Borneo still wear penis pins through their ampallang piercings, apparently to please the women. There are reports that women in Borneo say penis pins are to sex what salt is to food. However, the authors of *The Penis Inserts of Southeast Asia*, a monograph for the Center for South and Southeast Asia Studies, could find no direct quotes in the anthropological literature from any woman declaring her love for ampallang sex. The closest they get is a report that one woman said she preferred it when her husband wore one penis pin to when he wore three. They also note that a man in Borneo can use a penis pin with its ends sharpened to hurt or even kill a woman who makes him angry. In the West we don't have sharp-ended penis pins, and death by ampallang does not appear to be an option.

DICKS FULL OF PEARLS

Members of the Yakuza, the Japanese Mafia, decorate their bodies with beautiful tattoos, leaving the public parts—like faces and penises—bare. But they do decorate their penises if they serve time in jail, inserting pearls under the skin, one pearl for each year served. In *Modern Primitives,* Heather McDonald, a photographer who had a Yakuza boyfriend in Japan, describes the process: "They carve down a chopstick or toothbrush to a very sharp point, split the skin open about ¼" wide (anywhere from about ½" below the head to about ½" above the base), lift the skin up and away, insert the pearl, and then bandage it so the skin heals over and the area resembles a really big wart!"

Author Patricia Bosworth spent a few years in the 1970s as editor of *Viva,* the women's magazine that was published by *Penthouse. Viva* was the first women's magazine to run monthly photographs of totally nude men, and Bosworth, when she was editor, had to deal with the practice. She told me, "One guy came into the office, and he had pearls up the foreskin of his penis which supposedly made him a better lover. He came in with his manager—he had a manager for his penis. I didn't see his real penis; I saw photographs of his penis with the pearls, and it looked like he had pimples. We did not buy the photographs but *Playboy* did, eventually. He'd had the pearls inserted in Japan. I really was nonplussed. I mean, what can you say?"

CUSTOMIZED PENISES

PENIS TATTOOS

Years ago I knew a man with a tattoo on his penis, and one drunken evening he offered to show it to me. I turned him down, assuming that once he had it out he'd want to use it. Someone I know who did see the tattoo said it was just a bunch of scribbles. But whatever the design may be, when it comes to seduction a man with a tattooed penis has a talking point. I've heard about an Englishman alleged to have his coat of arms tattooed on his dick. Mad Dog, a famous San Francisco tattoo artist, told me he'd tattooed the words "your name" on the penis of one of his customers. This man wanted it so he could go into a bar and say to whomever he pleased, "I'll bet you I have your name tattooed on my dick."

Other penis tattoos Mad Dog has done include a lightning bolt, stars, hearts, cigar bands, rings, spirals. Some people with penis tattoos don't have any other tattoo work. "There seems to be not much rhyme or reason to it," he said. We were talking on the phone. He spoke slowly and sounded as if he'd never do anything to hurt you, a manner that must be soothing for his clients.

One man, he said, wanted his penis to be like a snake. "We covered it with a scaly pattern so it would look more reptilian, and then carried the reptile design on around his hip. And that worked out to be fairly interesting. On the head of the penis there were eyes; it's okay, but I don't think it's that convincing.

"Probably the oddest one was one person who wanted the head of his penis purple. He said he was intrigued by men whose penises are more naturally purple when they're erect, and he wanted his to be like that. So I said I thought he could do it quicker with a hammer. We spent a good deal of time mixing and coming up with the shade he thought he wanted."

Mad Dog said a penis tattoo doesn't hurt much unless it's on the head; tattoos on the shaft of the penis aren't any worse than ankle or shinbone tattoos. Even so, it's your *penis* that's hurting. The process could easily take a half hour—or much longer, depending on the complexity of the image—and then once it's done, it's done. Jewelry can always be removed, but there's no washing off a penis tattoo. Maybe for this reason penis-tattooing has not yet become a fad. Mad Dog, who caters in particular to the San Francisco gay community, estimated that penises accounted for only 2 percent of his business.

In New York I interviewed Dmitri Krylov at Kaleidoscope, a tattoo parlor on Canal Street. Dmitri had been recommended as one of the few tattooists in New York who was experienced with penises—and it turned out he had only done six. Polaroids of two of these were tacked up on the bright white walls, along with dozens of newly tattooed arms, shoulders, ankles and the odd breast or palm. One of Dmitri's penises had a tattoo of a penis on it. The other said, in bold black letters, VICIOUS. The rest, he told me, were done in Russia. They included a fly, a bee and a word that means something bad in Russian slang. He said his own penis was tattooed with the stamp of quality that appears on Russian merchandise. "When people see it they say, 'What is that?' and I can say, 'I was born that way.' Just for fun."

Penis-tattooing is not easy. The ointment tattooers normally use to wipe off excess ink makes a penis slip and slide around "like a piece of soap in the shower," Mad Dog said. He said he'd worked on erect and flaccid penises, and erections were the worst. But if a penis isn't erect—and usually they shrivel when the tattoo needle approaches—there's the problem of stretching the skin out so the tattoo will look right with an erection. Usually the client is enlisted as the stretcher.

Mad Dog (whose real name is Robert Roberts) told me this joke about penis tattoos. A man has a girlfriend, Wendy, whom he loves so much he gets her name tattooed on his penis. One day he's at his health club, and he sees a Jamaican man with what looks like the same tattoo. He approaches the Jamaican man and says, "Excuse me, I couldn't help noticing your tattoo. Do you have a girlfriend named Wendy, too?"

"What?" says the Jamaican.

"Your penis says Wendy on it, just like mine," says the first man.

"Wendy?" says the Jamaican. "No, mon. It says Welcome to Jamaica, Have a Nice Day."

BECAUSE IT'S THERE

So, why does a man tamper with his penis, or allow it to be tampered with? Sometimes it's to belong to a tribe. Sometimes it's to adorn himself. Sometimes it's for the sexual thrill. Whatever the reason, men who do something to alter the penises they were born with seem to feel more at home with themselves afterward. Before, they might have feared that someone else would harm it; instead they've hurt it themselves and found out they can take it. They've put their own mark on it, the way you might write your name inside a book.

PART
FOUR
THE SECRET
LIFE OF MEN

*T*his section is about sex and penises, and it represents my efforts to coax men into talking about it. The clearest information I got was from a few gay men, and from professionals who work with other men's penises (a urologist; a manufacturer of penis toys) or with their own (Richie Rich, a bisexual male hustler; Bill Margold, an X-rated video star).

One heterosexual man I interviewed alluded to the "mysteries of the penis," and then wouldn't speak of them—as if women who knew what men really thought and did with their dicks would no longer give them any respect. I think the opposite is true. The more I've found out about the secret life of men, the more sympathy I have for them.

CHAPTER TWELVE

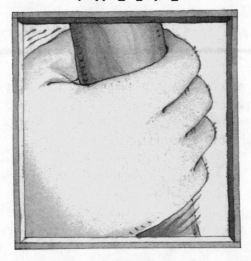

MASTURBATION

I had interviewed quite a few men about penises before illustrator Robert Richards gave me the lowdown.

Q: What are the mysteries of the penis?

A: I don't think it's a mystery. Men just don't want to talk about it. They don't want to talk about the fact they think about it day and night; they certainly don't want to talk about penis envy; they certainly don't want to talk about impotence, as related to themselves. I think men are very obvious. They're predators; they're ruled by their cocks. There's a theory that every forty-one seconds, or every thirty-eight seconds, or every minute and a half, a man has a sexual thought. I think that's true.

Q: You really think it's stronger than the mind?

A: I absolutely do. I think women don't understand the response men have to them on the street, because they're not men. Men don't need to be wooed; they see a woman and right away they have a rush, they feel something which is totally and directly related to their penises. Of course, construction workers have no right to holler at the women when they go by—but there is a kind of call of the wild about it, wolves baying at the moon.

Q: The penis has a mind of its own?

A: Yes. I think men masturbate more than women because it's less ritualistic, it's easy, it can be done in the most public of places. You can be having dinner with a man in a restaurant and he can go into the men's room and jerk off and come back.

Q: He would have to go into a booth to do that, right? He wouldn't do it at the urinal.

A: He might do it at the urinal if he was alone. He might even do it if there's another guy.

Q: Then that's a pickup.

A: It's a moment. Nothing more will happen. It's a moment. Now, I'm probably talking more about homosexual men than straight men, but I think it's all sort of equal. I really do think men are guided by their penises. Society refuses to deal with it and everyone wants to romanticize and intellectualize everything, but men are beasts. And maybe that's good. You have to have predators. In homosexual relationships, when I first came to New York, in my early twenties, things were so defined—there was the butch one and the femme one, the little girlie one and the big strong one. It was hideous. Now people are a bit more aware that if two men are together they're still both predators, and you have to really build a relationship around that fact. Because you're still going to have that construction-worker response, and it's not limited to construction workers. It doesn't arrive the day you get the job building the new Trump building. Okay, if you're well-bred you might not go "Pussy, pussy, pussy" when a woman walks by, but you might be thinking it.

Q: *That was very interesting what you said about jerking off in the men's room.*

A: It's extremely common. I think this has to do a lot with the accessibility of the penis. It's just one tug of the zipper away. You can be sitting with a man in a movie and he'll excuse himself and go to the men's room and by the time he comes back he's jerked off.

Q: *Are there other moments when a man might be doing that?*

A: At work it's very common. Certainly a tremendous amount of phone sex takes place on office phones. And apparently at any given moment there are thousands of people looking at pornography on the Internet.

Q: *They're looking at it, but are they jerking off to it?*

A: Of course they are. Guys are always jerking off. Don't take this lightly. If you get *Playgirl*, or *Penthouse*, a common letter will be from a woman who's caught her husband masturbating, and this will upset her no end. She'll say, "Aren't I satisfying him?" No. There isn't one person on earth who can satisfy any man. Men masturbate always. It's not a reflection on his relationship with his wife. He's shaving, and he suddenly thinks, I'll jerk off. And he does.

THE CASE AGAINST MASTURBATION

Much as men love masturbation, men in charge are always trying to make them stop. Christianity has been particularly severe about this. In the eighth century in Europe, when the Church published a series of penitential books describing sexual misdeeds and their penalties, masturbation got more space than any other sin.

Looking for a biblical justification, the Church found Onan, a figure from Genesis who was put to death for spilling his seed on the ground. Ever since, onanism has been a synonym for masturbation—though in fact Onan was not masturbating when he spilled his seed, he was practicing coitus interruptus. The law he broke was the one commanding him, after his brother's death, to beget a child with his brother's widow. Instead he was simply enjoying sex with his brother's widow. But this distinction must have seemed irrelevant. If you believe every ejaculation to be a fetus in formation, as the Church did, then a man who ejaculates for the thrill of it may be considered a murderer whether or not another person helps him out.

In Europe during the eighteenth and nineteenth centuries, when the pull of the Church was no longer so great, people found medical reasons to think masturbating was bad. All along men must have been secretly afraid that if they masturbated as much as they liked they'd never do anything else. Why else would they have believed so many bizarre theories about the evils of masturbation? In 1758 the influential Swiss doctor Simon-Andre Tissot published a book called *Onanism*, saying masturbation raised blood pressure inside the skull, damaging the nervous system and causing insanity. The American physician and signer of the Declaration of Independence, Benjamin Rush, was also convinced that masturbation caused insanity, or so he said in his 1812 work, *Medical Inquiries and Observations upon the Diseases of the Mind*. This view was accepted in some quarters up until the 1930s.

In 1882 *The Secret Sins of Society,* by An Old Practitioner, had this to say about masturbators: "Our insane asylums and poor-houses are crowded with these wretched victims. We have watched them in their drooling idiocy, a mere mass of corrupted flesh in the semblance of a man. . . . One man at the age of forty, who had reduced the sexual organs to a mere flabby rudiment, by this vice, sought a livelihood by buying and hauling dead hogs to a soap factory. Another, hump-shouldered, lop-sided, blear-eyed, drooling and filthy, carted swill to feed a few swine."

The Old Practitioner gave advice for detecting masturbators: ". . . a mawkish, shamed, repellent look is the surest sign." And, "As bad as the physical conditions are, the moral degradation is worse. The characteristics are the loss of memory and intelligence, morose, an unequal disposition, indifference to pleasures and sports, mental abstractions, stupid stolidity, etc."

According to Hoag Levins, in *American Sex Machines,* ". . . throughout the latter half of the 1800s . . . medical professionals organized national anti-masturbation movements that urged family members and peers to spy on and expose suspected masturbators."

But disapprobation had little effect on those determined to masturbate, and some of their guardians turned to mechanical means to try and stop them. Among the devices invented to prevent masturbation and registered by the U.S. Patent Office were: an abdomen-mounted anti-erection penis ring that drove sharp metal points into a penis that tried to expand while wearing it (1897); a wired harness that sounded a bell and delivered an electric shock if a penis became erect (1903); a mechanical penis sheath that locked (1906); and, for asylum wear, garments with crotches made of metal (1908), and impenetrable rubber-

and-canvas suits (1915). Similar devices were invented and sold in France, Germany and England.

It seemed that nothing could eradicate the epidemic of so-called self-abuse. Men kept masturbating. In *Sexual Behavior in the Human Male,* which drew its conclusions from thousands of interviews conducted during the 1930s and '40s, Alfred Kinsey announced that 92 percent of American men had masturbated to orgasm at some point in their lives. Some adolescent boys, he said, masturbated more than three times a day, with no ill effect.

Kinsey's writings helped to bring on the sexual revolution of the 1960s. In its aftermath, almost half a century later, many people masturbate and believe it's good for their health. Modern sex books are apt to point out its positive aspects. As Bernie Zilbergeld enumerates them in *The New Male Sexuality*: It's fun; you don't have to look your best; it teaches you what you like and you can share this information with your partner; if you're monogamous, it's a way of satisfying yourself when your significant other is not available; you can use it to overcome certain sexual problems.

In *The Hite Report on Male Sexuality*, published in 1981, men told Shere Hite that they were less inhibited sexually when they masturbated than they were having sex with a woman. Also their orgasms were stronger, because they could have them just as they chose, without any pressure to perform.

But even though it's not taboo anymore, men don't want to talk about masturbation. Psychosexual counselor Eva Norvind told me about treating sex offenders in prisons. "They blush if I talk about masturbation," she said. "They cannot talk about things like that. They can do all those sex crimes, but when I would bring up masturbation they would say, 'How can I say these words in front of a woman?'"

CIRCLE JERKS

Many of the men I interviewed told me a friend first showed them how to masturbate. Some of them participated regularly in circle jerks. These events were especially popular in the days before there was *Playboy,* or *Inches,* or the porn video. The boys would sit around in a circle, jerking off together, competing to see who could ejaculate first. It takes no time at all in that atmosphere, I was told.

According to Kinsey, most American men, when masturbating, like to climax as soon as they can, "which means it does not ordinarily continue for more than a minute or two. Some males, indeed, are able to achieve orgasm quite regularly in a half minute or so, sometimes in ten or twenty seconds."

With training like this, some men end up needing to be countertrained. Eva Norvind, who before she took up counseling was a Mexican B-movie star and a dominatrix, told me, "There are men who constantly masturbate, who masturbate three or four times a day. I try to teach these men abstinence can be terrific because it's not just about having an orgasm, but about the quality of the orgasm. You have the hamburger orgasm, the everyday thing, and you have the more special one, and it's good to abstain sometimes just to build up to that bigger something for another moment."

Some men are members of adult circle jerk organizations. At their meetings the men sit in a circle and jerk themselves off. The idea in this case is to prolong the experience as much as possible before finally ejaculating.

JACKING WITH JACK

The gay pinup magazine *Inches* has a masturbation columnist who calls himself Jack. Readers send Jack accounts of their masturbation fantasies to turn on other readers. But the most entertaining part of the column must be Jack's style of address: "Hey there palm-jockeys—and welcome back to Jack's Wonderful World of Wank!" is the way he starts one column. "Like usual I got a fistful of greasy jerk tips and JO memoirs to share with you horndogs. So 'get a grip' and get set to let loose some major loads this month—I sure as hell did. Fact is, I been wanking so much while writing this column that my hairy nads are running on empty. So let's get the balls rolling with a fan letter." Later in the column he reacts to a letter with a boot-licking motif: "I always enjoy some horndog licking on my boots while I sit back and crank my meat—especially if he tongues his way up to my balls while he's at it. There's few things better than a hot tongue scrubbing your cum spuds while you fire off your gravy." And later there's a tale of soldiers going at it: "Jeez Louise, just the thought of that spread-eagle soldier-hole had my lap-lizard so swole up I had to spank it till it puked all over my goddam belly." The man is a wanking poet.

FUN WAYS
TO MASTURBATE

INTERNET MASTURBATION SITES

Two good masturbation sites on the Internet are Jackin-World and the Masturbation Home Page. JackinWorld caters to beginning masturbators with pages of reassuring instructions: Wet or Dry? What Should I Be Doing With the Other Hand? How Fast Should I Go? How Tightly Should I Grip? And so on. It also supplies correspondents with topics to write about. For example: What household items or substances have you used to help you to masturbate? Some of the answers: Ziploc bags filled with warm water to simulate a woman's insides; pillows; the cardboard cylinder from a roll of toilet paper or paper towels; a sock; a bar of soap with a hole cut in it; and anything else that has a hole. Often lubricated plastic bags were used in between the penis and the hole. Among the lubricants: peanut butter; potting soil; motor oil ("It leaves behind a very nice smell, and my penis is very soft after I wipe it off"); chocolate sauce; warm honey. One fourteen-year-old boy said he used the toilet seat ("I get on my knees with the lid up, put my penis on the toilet, and lower the lid on top of my penis. With my penis between the toilet and the lid, I can 'hump' the toilet until I ejaculate into it."). A nineteen-year-old said he cut off one end of an eggplant, carved a hole, filled it with baby oil. "It helps," he said, "if the eggplant is cooked."

One man's letter to the Masturbation Home Page begins, "Reading this homepage makes me realize how normal I am—seems as if most guys have tasted their own cum, fucked pillows, etc." One wrote about his fascination with vacuum cleaners: "I've been using the vacuum cleaner on my penis for some years and I really love it. . . . Now when I've moved away from my parents to an apartment of my own I've been using my vacuum cleaner on my penis at least four times a week. . . . It's a great feeling when you feel the suction around the penis just as you're about to cum and then when the sperm get sucked into the bag."

Another man recommended an athletic form of masturbation—pointing one's penis straight up toward the belly button and securing it there with tight underwear or a Speedo bathing suit, then hanging from a door or door frame and opening and shutting the legs as if making a snow angel. Eventually, he said, "the tension that you are feeling will start to cause a tightening sensation in your cock. As you increase the movement of your legs, a feeling of 'wanting to cum' will start emanating from your cock. Suddenly the overwhelming build-up of tension will become too great and you will have an awesome orgasm without ever really touching your dick!"

AUTOEROTIC ASPHYXIA

Among the strange penis stories Enrique liked to tell me, some of his favorites were about men who went so far out for their orgasms that they ended up hanging themselves. The medical term for masturbation at the end of a noose is autoerotic asphyxia, and the point seems to be to scare yourself rigid. You're supposed to come near death and stop yourself in time, and meanwhile the lack of breath is causing light-headedness, while the fact that you just may die, and it's up to you to control the situation, is causing euphoria. Presumably you ejaculate while hanging.

One reason this method is so exciting is that accidents do happen. The movie *The Ruling Class* opens with an eccentric English lord, dressed in a tutu and getting his rocks off by near-hanging, whose chair falls down. Not too long ago three boys in New Jersey were found hanged in an attic. It wasn't a triple suicide—they noosed themselves for the sexual thrill, and the table they'd been standing on fell over at the wrong moment. When the Australian rock star Michael Hutchence, of INXS, died in 1997 by hanging himself with a belt, there were rumors he'd actually been up there trying to give himself a bit of pleasure. (The coroner, however, ruled the death a suicide.)

In a section on autoerotic asphyxia in the *Encyclopedia of Unusual Sex Practices*, author Brenda Love says, "Very little is known about people who practice asphyxia because most do not seek therapy and do not otherwise come to the attention of the medical profession unless they die." It's estimated, Love says, that from 250 to 1,000 men die from autoerotic asphyxiation each year.

AUTOFELLATIO

To judge from my recent party conversations, a great many men are interested in autofellatio. And why not? Its advantages are obvious. Who could possibly give a man a better blow job than himself? He could figure out just what pleased him, and do that. He could come before his jaw began to ache. He could decide whether he wanted to swallow or not, and no one would feel guilty about it.

Autofellatio, according to Kinsey, "is a common means of masturbation among rhesus monkeys, the macaque, mandrill, chimpanzees and other primates . . . and occurs quite widely among mammals of many other groups." But for most humans it remains merely a consummation devoutly to be wished. Kinsey says that many of the interviewees in his study said they'd tried to go down on themselves, but only two or three in a thousand were capable. The easiest way for a man to do it is to lie on his back and flip his legs over his head. And even that's not easy, unless he has a long penis and a flexible back. According to Brenda Love, those who practice autofellatio are split about the matter of ejaculation. Some like to swallow, some like the way their come feels on their skin, some like to listen to it as it whizzes past their ears.

157

CHAPTER

THIRTEEN

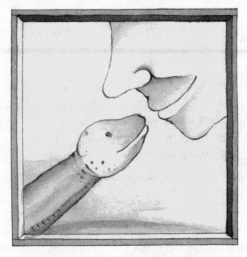

FELLATIO

If stand-up comics are to be believed, American hetero-sexual men can't get enough of fellatio. Some men whose wives or girlfriends won't satisfy their yearning go to pros-titutes for blow jobs. X-rated videos are made with the male desire for oral sex in mind.

When I asked the X-rated star Bill Margold about all the blow jobs in X-rated videos, he said, "The primary rea-son this industry exists is what I call the Vicarious Revenge Motif. We are a vicarious cathartic revenge for all the men who couldn't get the cheerleader when they were in high school, and never had a beautiful woman hanging on to the head of their dick." This traditional male view of fellatio—that the person performing it has been one-upped by the person on the receiving end—may have something to do with the traditional female reluctance to be a performer.

So I was glad when Dr. Jed Kaminetsky—who is a sex therapist as well as a urologist—described fellatio to me as more of a win/win situation. He said, "Oral sex is something that all men want. It feels good and also there's no pressure and no performance anxiety, it's just pure pleasure. Men always want to please their partner and delay orgasm, but here their partner is happy if they come quickly. Also, for most of the time the man is initiating, or he's much more active, and in oral sex he can just be much more receptive."

Fellatio also gives a man a visual treat, as one woman pointed out to me. "I've never performed oral sex and not had a man tell me he liked watching," she said. "When a woman is being given oral sex, all she can see is the top of a man's head. So it's not really a visual experience. But a guy sees something extremely sexual going on right in front of him."

Gay men are luckier than straight men when it comes to receiving oral sex. According to the 1981 *Hite Report on Male Sexuality*, the most recent survey of its kind, oral sex is the "most popular form of sexual activity" among gay men. On the other hand, many of the men who participated in the *Hite Report* who got their blow jobs from women were concerned that the women didn't really like doing it.

Helen Lawrenson published a merry piece in *Esquire* in the 1970s about her attempts, in the 1930s, to learn to make oral love. She and a few of her friends, she says, went at it studiously. "We keep practicing in a dogged way," she says she wrote to a friend, "although it is getting pretty hard to get any men to practice on, we are so terrible." She describes fellatio as "an acquired taste, like oysters."

Nowadays the practice of fellatio is much more wide-spread than it was when Lawrenson was first learning, then writing, about it—and its rise in popularity seems to have coincided with a parallel rise in the popularity of cunnilingus.

In my admittedly unscientific sample, all the women I interviewed said they liked giving oral sex sometimes, and most said when they did it they swallowed the semen. None of them said they liked the texture or taste of semen. "The taste doesn't bother me so much as the coating it puts in your mouth that you can't get rid of," one said. "I've had two long-term lovers, and with both I started swallowing because they asked. At first I didn't think I could. But after a while it was almost ritualistic and it became pleasurable for me to do it for him."

One said she had stopped swallowing because she didn't think it was nice for a man to see her gag on it. She said she believed men who were hard-core meat-eaters had worse-tasting semen than vegetarians. A meat-eater's come, she said, tasted "acrid, extremely bitter, the way you would imagine battery acid tastes." Another agreed. "I love giving oral sex," she said, "but I think any woman has to be hot to do it. Otherwise a cock just looks like a piece of kielbasa. And it's going to squirt you with battery acid and you know it. You're praying to get it over with, but you don't want the battery acid."

(Dan Anderson and Maggie Berman, authors of *Sex Tips for Straight Women from a Gay Man*, claim most gay men don't swallow. If they did, they'd miss out on the superior thrill of watching a penis ejaculate.)

It seems to me oral sex is more intimate than inter-course, because it requires you to go beyond pure rutting. You take a leap of faith, putting somebody's penis in your mouth. It doesn't make a perfect fit, the way it does, say, with a vagina. You need to use your imagination to engage with it. Luckily, humans have imagination. Animals don't, and you never see an animal giving head to another animal.

But ideas change. A report in the *New York Times* in April 1997 said teenagers were now engaging in oral sex as a less intimate and less risky alternative or prelude to intercourse. A fifteen-year-old girl was quoted: "For the people I know, sexual intercourse is a humongous thing. It's risky, and it's a big deal. But oral sex doesn't seem like sex. People may see the first time as a rite of passage, but after that, it's nothing much." It was reported that a nurse at Hunter High School in New York had begun stocking mint-flavored condoms without spermicide, labeled "ONLY for Oral Sex," next to the regular condoms. The mint condoms were flying off the shelves. The nurse told the *Times*, "In talking with kids, I found that a lot of them didn't think oral sex was sex. They think of it as a safe way of being close."

So in the winter of 1998, when President Clinton declared under oath that he hadn't had a sexual relationship with the White House intern Monica Lewinsky—though in fact she'd been an eager purveyor of presidential blow jobs—he was expressing a view that most New York teenagers could understand.

ADVANCED FELLATIO

According to several published descriptions, a good repertoire of basic blow-job techniques would include licking, sucking, blowing, humming and slipping the lips up and down the penis shaft while keeping the throat open for penetration. Some advanced practitioners use liquid aids for heating, cooling and keeping the penis alert, as if it were a fevered child. An expert might sip a bit of ice water or mouth a few ice chips when the penis is hot and hard enough, perhaps following up with a bit of warm coffee or cocoa. Champagne or mint toothpaste or Pop Rocks are recommended to make a stiff cock tingle.

Sometime in 1997 a story about Altoid mints and blow jobs was posted on the Internet, and it's still in circulation. It reads like the work of an Altoids copywriter—but may well be what it purports to be, a bemused account by a man who works for a technology firm. "Had the most interesting conversation with the top sales weasel at our company today," it starts out. "She came into my office and noticed I had a box of Altoids on my desk." This female sales weasel tells the narrator she's discovered by accident that chewing Altoids before you begin makes for an extraordinary blow job. The story of her finding has spread like wildfire around the office, with the result that "Having a box of Altoids on your desk is now like being part of the Secret Blowjob Goddess Society." (Altoids, the writer concludes, leave "a lasting tingle that is apparently quite exquisite." I've also heard that eating them temporarily increases the mouth's supply of saliva.)

Altoids gained further notoriety when they showed up in the Starr Report on President Clinton and the Monica Lewinsky affair. It's November 1997 and Monica is experiencing growing frustration in her attempts to be with the President. One late afternoon she manages to make her way into the Oval Office, where we get a tiny slice of love life on the run: "She also showed him an email describing the effect of chewing Altoid mints before performing oral sex. Ms. Lewinsky was chewing Altoids at the time, but the

President replied that he did not have enough time for oral sex. They kissed and the President rushed off for a State Dinner with President Zedillo."

Commerce being what it is, some New York drugstores now happily acknowledge the fellators among their customers, stacking Altoids next to the condom display.

CHAPTER
FOURTEEN

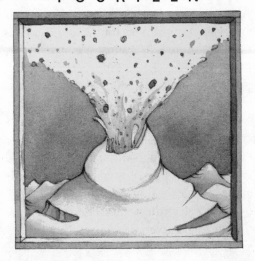

EJACULATION:
PRO AND CON

Men may think about sex every half minute, but at the same time they worry that sex may not be good for them. They're afraid it may deplete their vital juices, or distract them from the task at hand, or they think that because it's outside of wedlock it's a sin. In ancient Rome, where it was believed that sex was bad for the physical well-being and particularly the voice, musicians and actors and possibly athletes as well were infibulated. Their foreskins were pierced on each side and a ring put through so the foreskin would cover the glans at all times. They could urinate but could not get an erection.

In Victorian England infibulation was sometimes used as a cure for masturbation.

THE SECRET LIFE OF MEN

Frank Harris, the Victorian rake, says in his autobiography, *My Life and Loves*, that he learned of the virtues of abstinence when he was in his thirties and had himself circumcised as a prophylactic against syphilis. Afterward, recuperating in Heidelberg, he found erection painful and discovered that "absolutely complete chastity enabled me to work longer hours than I had ever worked: it was impossible to tire myself; in fact, I was endowed, so to speak, with an intense energy that made study a pleasure and with a vivid clearness of understanding such as I had never before experienced. At first I thought there must be some virtue in the climate; but one wet-dream made me realize that the power was in the pent-up semen."

Victorian Englishmen would say they were "spent" after they ejaculated, as if drawing on a limited bank account. The association of ejaculation with exhaustion is still with us. Folk wisdom has it that athletes should not have sex before the big game. On the other hand, if you ask a Western urologist he'll say a man ought to ejaculate at least once a week to keep his prostate healthy.

MULTIPLE ORGASMS FOR MEN

In the West we assume that men have sex in order to ejaculate. In the East the thinking is somewhat different. The ancient Chinese, who produced the world's earliest sex manuals, believed that sexual intercourse was, among other things, an important way of achieving harmony with nature. Like Westerners they felt uneasy about ejaculation, yet that was no hindrance, since they'd discovered how a man could have orgasms often, and ejaculate seldom.

EJACULATION: PRO AND CON

The Multi-Orgasmic Man, by Mantak Chia and Douglas Abrams Arava, lays out the Tao of sex for modern Americans. Patiently the book explains that orgasm and ejaculation are not the same thing. Ejaculation is a two-stage process, and a man can feel the delicious orgasmic contractions of stage one without proceeding to stage two and its debilitating depletion. As long as he doesn't ejaculate, he can keep having orgasms. They quote the ancient *Discourse on the Highest Tao Under Heaven*: "If a man has intercourse without spilling his seed, his vital essence is strengthened. If he does this twice, his hearing and vision are made clear. If three times, all his physical illness will disappear. The fourth time he will begin to feel inner peace. The fifth time his blood will circulate powerfully. The sixth time his genitals will gain new prowess. By the seventh his thighs and buttocks will become firm. The eighth time his body will radiate good health. The ninth time his life span will be increased."

During the first phase of ejaculation semen is produced in the urethra. According to Taoist theory, if a man can go that far and no farther, the semen will be reabsorbed into his body, enriching it with sexual energy. Other techniques circulate this sexual energy. "Self-cultivation," described by one multiorgasmic man as "somewhere between masturbation and meditation," is part of the training. A man who can cultivate himself for more than fifteen or twenty minutes without ejaculating can have intercourse for as long as he wants.

The goal is "whole body orgasm," which another multiorgasmic man describes as "more subtle, complete, satisfying. The whole process is not a feeling of a short explosion but of a longer and slower implosion. I don't feel empty afterward, which is easy to understand because with an explosion something leaves your body, but with an im-

167

plosion you still have it with you. There remains a deep satisfaction on the physical, emotional, and spiritual levels, which stays sometimes for hours, sometimes for days."

Tantra, a discipline developed in India around 5000 B.C., also views sex as a spiritual practice. In *The Art of Sexual Ecstasy*, Margo Anand explains, "Shiva was worshiped as the embodiment of pure consciousness in its most ecstatic state, and Shakti as the embodiment of pure energy. The Hindus believed that through uniting spiritually and sexually with Shiva, Shakti gave form to his spirit and created the universe. Tantra, therefore, views the creation of the world as an erotic act of love."

The Tantric view of sex is the obverse of the Christian. In Christianity, sex should only be used for procreation. In Tantra, sex for pure pleasure, because it feels so heavenly, is a way of worshiping god.

In *The Art of Sexual Ecstasy* breathing and imaging techniques are used to enhance intimacy, pleasure oneself, delay ejaculation. "There are many advantages to making love without ejaculation," Anand says. "For men, you can enjoy making love more often, and you will not feel depleted. When you *do* ejaculate after containing your energy longer, your orgasm is stronger. Because you will maintain an erection for a longer time, you can satisfy a woman more completely, bringing her through several intense orgasms. This will allow her to trust you more fully. She will feel your heartfelt desire to fulfill her. In return, you are sure to receive her unconditional love and experience a more harmonious relationship."

Both books refer to the practices described as sexual healing. One way in which they sound like healing is that they take the emphasis off performance. Most of the exercises can be done alone or with a partner, with or without an erection.

Workshops in Taoist and Tantric sex are currently available to those who seek them. I predict they'll become wildly popular as soon as someone figures out how to make complicated, spiritual sex lessons sound sexy.

WAYS TO DELAY EJACULATION

For those who are less spiritually inclined, here's a note from *Burton: Snow upon the Desert*, a biography of Sir Richard Burton by Frank McLynn: ". . . the object in all sexual intercourse is to delay the orgasm of the man and hasten that of the woman. To this end the Hindus employed all manner of techniques for preventing muscular tension. The essence of the 'retaining art' is to preoccupy the brain. Hindu males therefore used to drink sherbet, chew betel-nuts and even smoke during coition itself."

American men who want to delay ejaculation are most likely to think about baseball scores.

Aly Khan, famous as a lover during the mid–twentieth century, used to dip his elbows in cold water to keep himself from popping too soon. At least that's what Enrique told me. He said he'd heard it from someone who knew. He couldn't say, though, whether this method was employed before the act began, or during the course of it.

CHAPTER

FIFTEEN

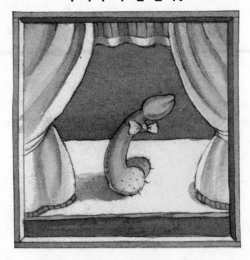

PENIS
ENTERTAINMENTS

If you enjoy watching penises, and live in a major American city in 1999, it's easy enough to see male strippers.

In New York you can see male strippers without even leaving your home, by tuning in to the public access cable channel 35 at the right time. The entertainment on this channel, late at night and early in the morning, consists almost exclusively of commercials for phone sex and escort services. The commercials come on one after another —women with inflated breasts offering them to the camera; men stepping forward, cocks at attention; so-called chicks with dicks, who display both breasts and cocks, for the person who wants everything. In between commercials, live strippers sometimes appear, and are interviewed about their new videos as if they were authors on a promotional tour. I personally find the male strippers' acts disappointing. They take it off, bit by bit, some of them with a great deal of flair, but when they get to the main event, the unveiling of the penis, the penis is always limp. Quite possibly I'm out of it, and limp dicks are exactly what most people are tuning in to see. But according to one of my informants, things used to be different on Channel 35 before a law was passed forbidding these strippers to touch their members.

CHIPPENDALE'S

Chippendale's was a sensation when it started out in 1978, as a nightclub where men stripped for women. Now the show tours the world, and in New York it can be seen at one club or another on Saturday nights only. Though it's no longer a novelty, it still gives the audience a thrill.

What you notice first when you enter Chippendale's is that all the men in the room have beautifully developed upper bodies. You notice because they're guiding you to your seat and acting as waiters, and they're naked from the waist up. Around their wrists they wear white French cuffs and around their necks white formal collars with black bow ties, so they look like rakish servants. They act that way too, eager to please and ever so courteous, clearly paying attention to you because you're a woman, and they appreciate women.

Most of the women who go to Chippendale's are in their twenties, and some are having bridal showers or bachelorette parties. (You can pick out the prospective brides because they wear bridal veils.) These women pay $50 each to sit at a table, or $40 for a folding chair in one of the rows behind the tables, to watch a striptease. And a tease it is. The show onstage celebrates women's desire to see some dick—by hiding it from them. No matter how much the women scream for it, dick is precisely what they never get to see, and everyone seems to like it that way. The dancers strip down to brightly colored G-strings; their dicks stir inside like hooded hawks. Or if a dancer takes his G-string off, as in a number done to Randy Newman's *You Can Leave Your Hat On*, he covers his dick with his hat. The women scream every time a dancer makes sexual motions—bumps, grinds, unzipping of flies, ripping off of undershirts; all these actions are greeted with gales of excitement. And it is exciting, in its very nice clean-cut way.

After a dancer does his number the emcee informs the already charged-up women that he's coming into the audience. The women stand up and wave dollar bills to show they want his attention. "Girls, don't miss out on Bobby V," the emcee will say. As Bobby walks among them the women stuff the bills in his G-string, or hand them to him for him to hand to a man who walks nearby, holding a money pouch. The dancers pay special attention to the women with the bridal veils, the ones celebrating their last night of freedom. But with all the women they keep their distance. They almost touch, or they lap-dance or dirty-dance for only a beat or two, or they get away with a kiss on the cheek if they can. I stood up to try to dance with one of them—he hugged me, took my dollar and said, "Thank you, baby."

Of course, some rude girls grab for the dick, but they don't get very far. The dancers are expert at slithering away, and they're accompanied by a cadre of naked-chested, black-tied bodyguards.

By the end of the show, which takes an hour and forty-five minutes, the women are up and dancing. The plastic glasses their drinks came in (you get two with the price of admission) lie tipped over on the floor. The waiters and ushers start mopping and piling up chairs while the girls are still having their pictures taken with their favorite Chippendale's stars.

THE BIG-DICK CONTEST

I took Enrique with me to a bar called King where they were supposed to have a big-dick contest at three one morning, but the contest didn't materialize. Instead there was a muscle-butt contest, during which six or seven men got up on a small stage and mooned the audience.

While we were sitting around at King, waiting for the wrong contest to begin, we watched another kind of penis entertainment. A thin, well-built man was quietly roaming the room, wearing nothing but black boots, red and white socks, a brown leather apron that covered the top third of his thighs, and a jockstrap. The jockstrap was obviously not in use at the moment; this man with the apron had a dick so big you could see his foreskin peeking out beyond the apron's bottom, and he wandered slowly from customer to customer, as if the weight he carried had him in a trance. Someone would call him over, stick some money in the strap of the jockstrap and shove a hand under the apron to cop a feel. Then he'd move on.

After all the customers had a chance at him, another man took his place. This one wore a towel around his waist, and boots and socks. People put money into his socks, then put a hand under his towel. Later I told this to a friend, who said she'd paid to feel up a guy who was walking around with a big dick inside a bikini at another club, called Escuelita. I said I thought only men did it. "I gave him a dollar and I put my hand inside," she said.

"That's the way it works." I asked her what it was like. She said, "It was long and thick, and I pinched it. He said, 'Ow, that hurts.'"

THE GAIETY

Just as heterosexual men go to topless bars to wonder at women's breasts, so do homosexual men go to male strip shows, for the cocks. The Gaiety, Manhattan's premier male strip theater, is open every day on Forty-sixth Street near Broadway. On Saturdays there are five shows, and at each one there are twelve acts. Men sit in silent rows, watching the stage, which is slightly elevated so everyone looks up at the strippers. There are signs on the walls saying "Absolutely No Sexual Activity Is Permitted." In the aisles, burly security men watch to make sure no sex takes place.

The strippers look like nice, clean-cut college boys. Each comes on to recorded music, and during the first song he teases. He might amble up and down the stage as if he were on his way to biology lab; then he might pull up his shirt and show his chest development, or take off his belt and flick it on the stage floor, or turn around and pull down his pants so the audience can see his nice butt. At the end of this number there's a break—the stage is empty, and everyone waits impatiently for the stripper to return. When he does he's naked, except for socks and running shoes, and his dick is erect. The erection stands out like a neon sign. Each erection gets applause—and most of them have flagged before the clapping stops. The men dance around with their disappearing erections, and customers put money in the socks.

This is how far gone I was in my penis research by the time I went to the Gaiety: I thought the show was sweet. The men were clean-cut, they were there to please, they strutted, but in a modest way. They weren't show-offs, though apparently they did enjoy being naked for us. I liked the way they were tender when they caressed themselves.

I told Enrique, who went with me, how sweet I thought it was. Enrique believes that at some early point in human history women used to get in heat and men used to line up to have sex with them. These men coming out erect one after another reminded him of the great primordial gang bang. He said, "It didn't seem sweet to me."

When we got tired of watching the penis parade we went to the lounge, to one side of the theater, where fruit punch and Cheetos are served, and the strippers meet customers and make assignations. Later I was told that the strip show doesn't pay them much. Their real career is hustling, and the strip show is the advertisement. On the whole, the men who engage their services don't want anything more than to adore their cocks or give them blow jobs. My informant said a fair number of the strippers are heterosexual. I asked him how that could be. "Oh, you know," he said, "men will fuck anything."

CHAPTER
SIXTEEN

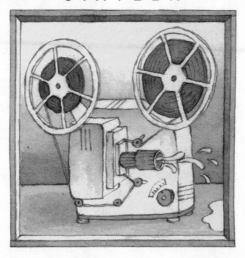

DICKS ON FILM:
AN INTERVIEW
WITH
BILL MARGOLD

Bill Margold is one of those stars of X-rated videos whom other men may envy. Margold calls himself "the leading authority on the X-rated industry in the world." He's performed in, directed, written and publicized X-rated videos and, in his mid-fifties, he still goes in front of the camera for the occasional masturbation scene. Mostly he functions as an industry activist—and gives advice to the performers through an organization called Protecting Adult Welfare, or PAW.

At the time I interviewed Margold he was living alone after a long relationship with Viper, a female X-rated star whom he called "the most exciting and magnificent person I've ever known." I phoned him at his house in Los Angeles, wanting to know his professional secrets. It was seven in the morning there, and he was alarmingly wide awake.

Q: *How did you get into this business?*
A: My degree is in journalism, and I got into the industry to start writing about it. I have written hundreds and hundreds of firsthand accounts of what it's like to be in front of the camera, underneath the camera, behind the camera and over the camera. I was very much a nerd as a child, and a toad. Until I became a journalist, in fact, I was quite introverted, but the minute I got a byline, I felt I had power, and with the power I began to explode and to move into all areas. Essentially, I came into an industry for which I've coined the term "Playpen of the Damned." I've lived everything everyone else dreams about on every level. I've done three hundred videos and films, I've done five hundred sex scenes, and yes, I have been in the trench using my dick as the shovel, many, many, many times. Some of my scenes are somewhat legendary. I do have a dick that ranks in the top one tenth of 1 percent—my dick's well over ten inches. And I did not know I had, I guess, a big dick until I was in bed with a woman who told me I did. She was surprised I had never compared my dick with anyone else's taking showers in gym class. But my dick doesn't show much interest until it gets erect. My erections are analogous to the kind the King used to get, because of course his was the biggest of all the dicks in the business.
Q: *The King. Do you mean Elvis?*

A: The King is John C. Holmes. I gave him his nick-name back in the seventies, and he was living proof that all men are not created equal. He was to the X-rated industry what Babe Ruth was to the baseball industry. He elevated it into national prominence. Because the King was someone that people looked at and said, Man, that's amazing. That was a big dick.

Q: *How big was that?*

A: It was over twelve inches. It was ominous-looking. His was the staff by which all other men were measured.

Q: *Being big is one thing; the other thing is being able to function. How do you get it to work on demand?*

A: Mind over matter. I don't let anybody touch me until I'm ready to work, because my left hand has been my best friend since I was thirteen years old and discovered the wondrous pleasures of masturbation. Basically from the moment I'm aware I'm going to do a sex scene I start playing with myself. I pull my dick away from my body, pulling it down, trying to interest it in getting an erection. The trick is to start suggesting to it that it's going to be going somewhere. The minute I start playing with my dick the end result—and I'm aware of that—is the release, which is the ultimate reason to get an erection, so that's what I'm looking forward to. Once my dick is big I can do whatever needs to be done with the female in the room.

I much prefer the oral sex scenes to the hard-core penetration, because my knees are pretty banged up from playing football and I'm a very clumsy man. The scenes that are easier for me are when I'm standing up and the woman is on her knees. That's also good for the image on camera; it sells—and, of course, I believe the most important sex scene we can bring to the public is the oral sex scene anyway. Because many men can go home and get laid but they might not be able to go home and get blown.

Q: Why do men like receiving oral sex so much?

A: Power. Absolute, total power. The man has nothing to do but to lie back and enjoy it. He has subjugated the woman into a situation where she is servicing him.

Q: And when the man services the woman?

A: Women are much more tied up in their orgasms than men are. They continually look for a Roman candle, when a firecracker would do. They're always waiting for the ultimate release, so they lock themselves up like walnuts and almost challenge the man to get them off. There's no challenge when a woman is working on me, because I can come whenever I want to. I can give you a come shot, or what is known as a money shot, in ten seconds. In fact, I invented the ten-second come shot in 1973; it's the standard for the industry. But let's get back to the psychodrama of sex, on camera or even off. I love going down on a woman, because there are all kinds of wonderful things down there you can play with. And you can feel women getting excited; you really have them at your mercy. Once you're locked in to their nerve center they lose control, and that is a treat.

Q: Isn't it the same the other way around, that the woman has the man at her mercy?

A: She doesn't, because any man who's in charge of his own dick should be able to go off when he wants to, not when she wants him to. However, in the vagina, that's where the man is in over his head, literally. Most men, once they're locked up in that cavern of pulsation, they get trapped in the lust of the moment. They think, Oh, now I'm getting laid, so this is the ultimate thrill. Oh, now I'm having so much fun, oh this is great, oh goody. And of course they lose complete control.

Q: So how do you control it?

A: I psych my mind out. In fact, I'm sort of mechanical. It's the least intimate part of the sexual act, as far as I'm concerned. Once you're in there, you're doing basically an animal act.

Q: What makes a female adult star good to work with?

A: Lesllie Bovee was a star of the 1970s and she was a beautiful brunette, very sexy, and her mouth was like an oven. That woman just had suction power. I had been told she was the best, and she was. She's not the best I ever had penetrational sex with; that was a woman named Danielle Martin. Having sex with her was like climbing into an oven. A full-blown roaster.

Q: Guys who are average size think guys who have big dicks have more fun.

A: More doesn't mean more. You gotta know what to do with the damned thing. There's a whole lot that's done before you even screw the woman when you have a real big dick, because you've got to prepare them for the penetration. I used to watch the King work, and he would knead the women like dough in order to get them ready for penetrating. The women all said he was an excellent lover. If you watch the King on camera you notice he's not jamming it in there; it's easy, it's gradual, it's comfortable-looking. He's not brutalizing their internal organs.

Q: Is your penis a separate entity with a mind of its own?

A: I think so. I do talk about it in another person. I'm very happy with him—he's a good-natured kid, he does what he has to, he's independent, and I will fulfill whatever he needs whenever he wants it.

Q: Why do you think your penis functions so well?

A: Maybe just the luck of the draw. I don't know my genetic makeup, being adopted. But I don't deny myself a release. If I sense there's a need for an ejaculation I will

181

have one. I don't wait until a better time to masturbate, I simply do it, and then I go on with my day. One of the few quotes I use that's not my own is a magnificent quote from Bernardo Bertolucci: "The true obscenity is not in the hands of the masturbator but in the hands of the person who spanks the hands of the masturbator."

Q: What are the disadvantages for guys whose dicks are their meal tickets?

A: They're hit men. It's the *High Noon* syndrome. To a certain extent the ones who are consistently good at it are bigger than life. They're as legendary in their own prowess as any professional athletes. I liken what we do, in baseball jargon, to bottom of the ninth, bases loaded, full count and you can't foul off a ball.

Q: Among the men you counsel, is the main problem getting hard and staying hard?

A: I've had very few of those people come and see me. The thing is, unless you're capable of doing it, very shortly in your career you'll no longer be performing. If you check the lineage of this industry you'll find out the same men have been around forever. The nature of this business begins with John C. Holmes, Harry Reems, Eric Edwards, Jamie Gillis, and on this coast Rick Cassidy and Ric Lutz. The most important one is Ron Jeremy, the Hedgehog. Ron Jeremy has a big dick. Ron Jeremy is living proof that anyone can get laid. I'm sure you've seen him. He's a furry-looking man. I gave him the name Hedgehog. And T. T. Boy. He's the best we have today. I am not famous for being a stud, because that's only one tenth of what I've done in this business. I was very lucky to do it, but that's not what I want to be remembered for. I prefer you remember the people like T. T. Boy and Tom Byron and Marc Wallice and Peter North and Joey Silvera and Paul Thomas and Herschel Savage, and Rocco, and Sean Michaels, and Ray

Victory, and Billy Dee; these are the ones who were the foot soldiers—or dick soldiers, for lack of a better term. These were the ones who got up, got in, got out, got off, when it counted.

Q: *Do guys in the porn business all have big dicks?*

A: No. They have functional dicks. It's more important to get it up than to have a size that doesn't function at all. Because the end result of what they're looking for is the ejaculation. The come-shot, desirably in the face.

Q: *Why?*

A: I believe that's the purest form of cathartic vicarious thrill revenge. I think a come-shot on the breast is worthless. I don't like tits. A come-shot on the belly looks like some sort of antipregnancy-method withdrawal.

Q: *I've heard that come is good for your skin.*

A: You come what you eat, basically. I think you'll find there's a wonderful curative purpose to what we ejaculate, if it's healthy. Viper, the woman I used to live with, demanded, on Saturdays after football, a come-shot in the face. She would scrub it into her face and leave it on until it dried and then peel it off, and you could see the dirt coming out. It took all the impurities out of her skin. Viper's skin was like a pearl.

Q: *When you ejaculate on camera, is it supposed to shoot far?*

A: A come-shot—they don't call it that because it just sort of dribbles out. It does shoot across. The best of all of them in this business for come-shots is Peter North. They call him the Beer Can, because of the explosion of the beer can.

Q: *But what's the big deal of having it shoot? Is it like a pissing contest?*

A: I think the end result of a good come-shot shows the pent-up amount of release, the explosion. A great come-shot just coats the woman's face. I've had some pretty good ones. My testicles are maybe the biggest in the history of this business. They're just enormous, and they hang a lot lower, and they're unusually heavy. I've never figured out what that's all about except that as a child, living relatively penuriously, I had loose-fitting clothing, so my testicles were allowed to develop and drop very low. Sometimes I have to pull them out of the way because they obliterate the angle. I have a feeling that makes for me a much more copious come-shot. You lose in elasticity as you get older, but I don't really care about that. The pleasure of the release is the ultimate reason you have the erection. It's a very very satisfying and unparalleled feeling.

CHAPTER
SEVENTEEN

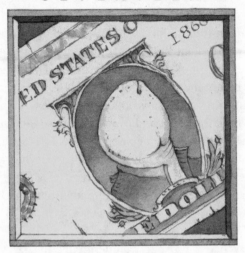

HUSTLING:
AN INTERVIEW
WITH
RICHIE RICH

"Richie Rich" has been working as a hustler for six years; his penis is the tool of his trade. He services both men and women, advertises in gay magazines and also gets clients through word of mouth. They get in touch with him by voice mail, and he goes to their apartments or offices. He has a slight build and he was wearing jeans, a T-shirt and a baseball cap when we met for lunch in a Greenwich Village luncheonette. He said I would recognize him because he looked like a teenager, but when I asked him later how old he was he said he wasn't a kid.

Q: I hear you have a big dick. Is size an advantage in your business?

A: Men hire me because I'm the size they want, specifically. Gay men know what a specific size is going to feel like, and look like. Women don't. They just know you're better endowed as opposed to less well endowed and that with you it's satisfaction guaranteed. But there are guys who know eight and a half as opposed to seven and a half as opposed to nine and a half. And that may have originated with them knowing exactly what they measure and they're an inch and a half short of what they'd like to be. As if they were going to have sex with themselves. It's kind of odd.

Q: What about shape?

A: When a prospective client calls me he wants to know, do you stick straight out, do you turn up, do you turn to the left. Some people want to be surprised, but most people want to know. I stick straight out. There are multitudes of men who prefer a slight curve up, and I will sometimes not get that appointment.

Q: Are there things about the penis that women don't know that you wish they did?

A: Yes. Certain women are afraid of it. They want it, but they don't know why they want it. But the more a woman delves and investigates what will turn men on, the more satisfying it will be for her. It's the same thing the other way around—when a man investigates he really knows how to turn a woman on and bring her to orgasm. He doesn't do it to please himself, but ultimately he does please himself because the more you turn a woman on the more excited you're going to be. You know what? If you bring a woman to a point where she has multiple orgasms, you will probably have multiple orgasms, if you just concentrate on what it's really doing to her. There's also a serious percentage of women who are interested in men's butts, and although they have regular intercourse their attitude says that's not the part of the body they really care about. Visually. And that comes across to a man very quickly.

Q: *Are women good at oral sex?*

A: I don't think they're as interested orally as men are, and even if they are interested they're not usually as good as men. They have less idea what something feels like, less idea what's happening to it than other men do.

Q: *You need to get erections on demand. How do you do it?*

A: That's tough. It takes a lot of technique. Sometimes it doesn't take any technique at all. What I'm very good at is finding my own fantasy. I can always do it once. When you get there the first time and it's physically not doing it for you, you're still working off the fact that you're getting paid—that they called you, they want you, they heard about you. But I already know if it's a lot of work it won't be worth it for me, or for them, in the long run. I already know at the first appointment there won't be a second appointment, and I'll give them a hundred and ten percent, and they'll be left with that memory. And that keeps the word of mouth going. That's better for me.

Q: *How many can you do in a day?*

A: The average is three a day. The maximum amount could be nine. It depends on which appointments.

Q: *Do you have to ejaculate each time?*

A: No. There are men who don't want that—specifically don't want that. It's for themselves to get off and they would prefer that you don't. That's when I can fit nine in.

Q: *That could be frustrating.*

A: It could be. But if you have nine appointments, it's not. You know eventually it's going to hit the mirror. So if I have two or three people who are in it for the hour and a half, and they expect it, then I know I can't do nine. It's got to be a couple of hours between appointments, there's got to be ginseng, there's got to be a nap, Häagen-Dazs. Those are my aphrodisiacs.

Q: Do you ever feel as if you're burning out?

A: No. I take lots of time off. I take long vacations, and I don't work every day. I keep a regular job so I have something tangible for the tax man. And I'm in acting school, I'm in plays, I work in films. Right now I probably make about sixty thousand dollars a year from my profession, and that means I only work three or four days a week when I work. If I worked five days a week twelve months a year I could make ninety thousand. And I practice only safe sex.

Q: Do you have a standard rate or does it vary?

A: It starts real low, ninety dollars, and goes to five hundred—or much more for a weekend. It depends on what they want. Some people want dinner, theater, sex. Some people just want you to come over, pull down your zipper and fuck them in the mouth for fifteen minutes and leave. In the afternoon, that's ninety dollars. I have a guy who works behind the counter in the post office. He calls me once a month, fifteen minutes and I'm out.

Q: Do you see this as an ongoing part of your life?

A: I don't want to do it much longer than another year. I hope my acting career will take off. If you don't put enough physical and spiritual energy into what you really want to do, you get lost.

Q: What else do you do for the health and vigor of the penis?

A: First and foremost I make sure I give it a rest. I use a special skin cream, by Kiehl's, a combination of that and baby oil. It's for sensitive skin—there's no lanolin, nothing in it that could sting or burn. I have a high-protein, high-carbohydrate, high-calorie, low-fat diet. Red meat, chicken, fish. I also take a designer protein shake twice a day. Diet does make a difference, I swear to you. The protein intake adds to your testosterone abilities; not to your sperm count, but it gives you a more powerful ejaculation. You even see a difference in color with high protein—it's lighter. People who drink a lot of alcohol take a lot of their vitamin C and protein out in urinating, and they'll have a clearer ejaculate.

Gaining energy there is also a matter of mental relaxation. You have to be able to transcend any bad feelings—that's a given for anybody sexually.

I also swim every morning. It's an exercise that puts no strain on the penis whatsoever. With other exercises, even walking, there's a gravitational pull. And patchouli oil, that's a spiritual thing with me; I put it up top and below. I think the odor, there, mixed with a man's odor, turns people on.

Q: *Do you have a separate private love life?*

A: Yes I do. Which of course we will not talk about.

Q: *Do you prefer men or women?*

A: Generally I prefer women, specifically I prefer men. The general stereotype of women I prefer. They're more sensitive, stronger, usually emotionally more intelligent—women who are in touch with themselves are really superior. Plus they can have a kid if they want to, just for the hell of it. But there are few women who live up to that. So specifically there are men I enjoy more, because they may have less substance but they're more in touch with it. And they happen to be gay, because I wouldn't have met them otherwise. There are some people I see who are pretty much heterosexual men, categorically they're heterosexual, and they don't interest me at all.

Q: *How do you feel about your penis?*

A: That's the part of my body I respect the most, and the part I know will get me through—if I have a hard time, if I have a good time, if I have a slow time, if I have a late time, I just know that's me, I'm a phallic kind of guy. I'm like, dick first, then there's the rest of me. I can walk down Eighth Avenue and—it's not protruding or sticking out, but people just seem to focus there. That's the part of my body that people want me for.

Q: *Do both men and women focus on you there, or more men?*

A: On the street? Men. But the real women who are in touch with themselves whom I see, they do like it, they like the fact that it's big and it's not dysfunctionally enormous, and it works. I pay no attention to it whatsoever when I'm with them. Gay men like it when you pay attention to your own penis. Women want you to pay attention to them. And when they want to pay attention to your penis, and play with you and fool around with you, they will.

Q: *Were you always very sexual?*

A: Always. To an extreme. Bisexual people probably always are. I think they learn about themselves younger. I came out of the closet when I was fourteen. I realized I was bisexual when I was seventeen. Once you realize you're bisexual it's really fucked up. I look at a lot more people sexually, I get in a lot more trouble, I'm indecisive about relationships. Other people don't know what to think.

Q: *Anything else about the way your life is your penis?*

A: I make decisions about what clothes to wear based on how I look there. I make decisions on what underwear to wear based on how I look there. I want to be suggestive to a certain extent, but not to be obvious. I wear my jeans loose. I'm totally into what I look like unerect as well. If I'm being photographed and they want it not erect it looks the best if I need to urinate. I'll have a six-pack of beer beforehand and hold it in, because whatever that does to the solar plexus, it makes it hang a little lower and wider even though it's soft. You don't get that "I'm cold" look around the penis. This is for real, I'm totally serious. Then the session can only go an hour and a half because that's about as long as I can hold it. If it's to be erect I handle that differently.

Q: The solar plexus. Do you do anything special for that?

A: I do about 160 Roman Chair sit-ups every morning. It helps to use a machine that holds your ankles in place. You sit up straight and lower your head all the way to touch the floor, isolating the lower abdomen so you release the lower back from pressure. If you don't work those muscles out regularly, if you can't flex them, you can't relax them. You have to be able to relax them in order to control what's happening with your penis.

Q: So are you in control of it or is it in control of you?

A: That's a good question. Probably a combination of both. In a lot of ways it's in control of me, but I'm enjoying it, so I'm in control of what level of enjoyment I'm getting out of it.

Q: Do you get unwanted erections, not connected with sex?

A: They are connected to sex, just probably on an unconscious level. I pick up a lot of subliminal messages, and some of them I actually get as real messages, because of what I do for a living. Because I find men and women interesting I think maybe I pick up more subliminal messages than most people. In some ways a person who thinks with his dick is more in touch.

Q: Is there an equation between sex and love for you?

A: Yes. When I'm servicing a client I don't have to fall in love with them but there are certain people I have a really good physical time with and I can lie in bed with them for

191

an hour afterward and talk to them about all kinds of things and there's a part of me that's falling in love with them, absolutely. My definition of falling in love. And I am right now in love with an enormous amount of people to a certain extent and for different reasons. You know, you get one heart.

CHAPTER

EIGHTEEN

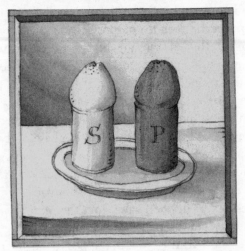

PENIS
PRODUCTS

Early humans must have discovered penis substitutes and extensions at about the same time they figured out that penises were sex organs. Penis substitutes are mentioned in the Bible and in ancient Indian and Chinese texts. Paintings of women using penis substitutes may be seen on Greek vases of the fifth century B.C. These dildos, known as *olisboi* (a word derived from a verb meaning to glide, or to slip), were usually made of wood or padded leather and were doused with olive oil before use.

Orthodox Hindus disapprove of dildos as "insults to Shiva, whose Lingam is ever-erect." Nevertheless the *Kama Sutra,* in the first century A.D., recommended things that could be used "in connection with or in place of the lingam." They could be made of "gold, silver, copper, iron, ivory, buffalo's horn, various kinds of wood, tin or lead, and should be soft, cool, provocative of sexual vigor, and well fitted to serve the intended purpose." Described, along with coverings to thicken the lingam and give it texture, are penis substitutes made of wood, gourd or oiled reeds that can be tied to the waist with strings.

The ancient Chinese used a great variety of sex aids, including substitute penises, penis caps, ribbons tied to the balls, and carved jade rings worn at the base of the penis with a protruding part that stimulated the partner's clitoris.

More recent Chinese and Japanese erotic drawings show women employing dildos to stimulate themselves and each other. In one I saw, from the Ming dynasty, a woman lies reading a book. One ankle rests on the opposite knee. She's wearing a dildo strapped to the other ankle, and using it to masturbate. Enrique told me he once saw a photograph of a jade dildo that had belonged to a Japanese naval officer's wife during World War II. At the flat end it had a locket, and inside the locket was a photograph of the woman's husband in his naval uniform. "It was very pretty because the jade changed color," he said, "and I guess you could call it romantic, that she would think of her husband when she pleasured herself."

MODERN DILDOS

Most of today's dildos aim not for romance but for verisimilitude, and instead of precious materials they're made of moldable plastic, latex or silicone. In a modern American sex-toy store they make an impressive display—shelves and shelves of lifeless but fleshy penises, like one small section of a vast phallic arsenal. Dildos are used by both men and women, both to masturbate and to have sex involving more dicks than there are people with dicks in the room. They're available in all sizes, from three inches to several feet, with or without balls. Some are constructed at the base so you can suction them to the bathroom wall, or the floor, or whatever surface turns you on. Or a woman can buy a dildo with a harness. Another alternative is a double dildo. A woman can put one end inside of her and with the other end pretend to have one of her own. Or two men can use one to abut each other, back to back. Dildos come in a variety of skin colors as well as in luminous pastels. Some have pumps attached, and get bigger when you pump them up. Some are more realistic than others, and the most realistic of all are molded from the dongs of real men. Among all dildos, the ones molded from the dongs of porn stars are the best sellers.

Phil Berman, of Flip Manufacturing, Inc., figures he was the first to mold the penis of a porn star, but at the time he was working for a sex-toy company that wouldn't manufacture and sell such a thing. This company made dildos, but considered a dildo that realistic-looking to be pornographic.

So before Berman could start his own company and get his Rex Chandler and Tony Montana dildos out, Doc Johnson Enterprises released the Jeff Stryker. The Jeff Stryker is the best-selling dildo of all time—perhaps because Stryker is a star in both homo- and heterosexual X-rated videos. Eventually Stryker sued Doc Johnson, which was making money, he said, using his dick in ways he hadn't authorized and was not getting paid for. The case was carried on Court TV; at one point the judge had a lineup of dildos on his desk and he challenged Stryker to pick his member out of the bunch. Stryker did, of course, winning the right to use his name and his penis. Doc Johnson also retained the right to use it.

Like Cynthia Plaster Caster, Berman said he uses "a dental formula" to make his molds. "We do this in my office. There are no aesthetics to the room, though the lights are dimmer than I would normally work with. But we're talking about professionals who work with their penis for a living. We just have the actor get an erection—he might have his partner with him to help do that, or we might bring someone in. Then the partner applies the material—it keeps the erection going much more easily than if I were to go over there and slap some plaster on his penis."

Some of Berman's other popular products are the Jurassic Cock and the Cock-a-Doodle Douche. Jurassic Cocks are soft, rubberlike sculptures that are phallic in size and shape but designed to look like dinosaurs—and they're legally for sale in areas where dildos are still illegal. The Cock-a-Doodle Douche is an actual douche kit with an applicator in the shape of a penis.

Sex-toy stores are filled with such penis novelty items, some of which have very little apparent connection with the sex act—penis salt and pepper shakers, penis soap on a rope, penis chocolates and so on.

COCK RINGS

At The Leather Man, in the heart of Greenwich Village, where they sell aids and accessories for every imaginable sort of sexual activity—gay, straight and other—cock rings are the most popular items. Cock rings get pulled over the cock and balls to lie flat against the pelvis, and most people who use them believe they prolong erections by restricting blood flow. But Robert Hansen, a cock-ring salesman at Leather Man, put it this way: "It's hard to say they make the erection last longer, because their main function is to increase sensation. They restrict the blood flow very slightly. They make the cock a teeny bit harder for a teeny bit longer, which also increases sensation. Also, men wear them under a tight pair of jeans because it's the Wonderbra for a penis. It pushes out and presents."

Rings come in small (1½" diameter), average (1¾") and large (2"). There are two main types, the solid ring and the leather strap that fastens with snaps, buckle or Velcro. "To some men the idea of a solid ring around everything is a little frightening," Hansen said to me. "But if you can get it in, you can get it out. It will always relax if you just wait. You know the story that there are alligators in the sewers under New York City. It's the same with the story about someone who knows someone who had to go to the hospital to have a cock ring removed. I don't believe it because I've never met that person."

Dr. Jed Kaminetsky has met more than one of those people. "They put these constricting rings around their penis and scrotum, fell asleep and left them on for twelve or twenty-four hours and their penis is all blown up. Sometimes it can be hard to get the ring off if it's too swollen," he told me. "But usually the swelling will go down once it is taken off. You just use heat, and sometimes antibiotics."

In the gay community cock rings are also used as bracelets and key rings, and a chrome cock ring is often hung on a chain around the neck. In 1993, Mattel toys manufactured a hip version of Barbie's boyfriend Ken, called Earring Magic Ken, and he wore what looked just like a chrome cock ring on a chain. When questioned by reporters, the Mattel people pleaded innocence—they were simply following fashion. But gay men noticed, and that may be why Earring Magic Ken was, according to Mattel, "the best-selling Ken doll ever."

CHAPTER

NINETEEN

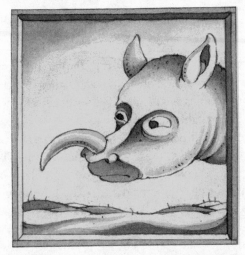

IMPOTENCE

When it comes to sex, people can fake almost anything —interest, surprise, amazement, passion, orgasm. The one thing no one can fake is an erection, and this puts men in an awkward position. They're the big, strong sex, and yet their temperamental penises can bring them low.

In 1968, when *Playboy* asked sex therapists Masters and Johnson the chief cause of impotence, Masters answered, "Fear. Regardless of why or under what circumstances the male fails to achieve or maintain an erection the first time, the greatest cause of continued sexual dysfunction thereafter is his fear of nonperformance."

(In this way impotence is somewhat similar to Koro, an epidemic condition that breaks out sporadically, mostly in the Far East, mostly among ethnic Chinese. Koro's only symptom is a conviction that one's penis is retracting into one's abdomen. To halt the regression, afflicted men have tied their penises to their legs; they've used clamps, chopsticks, clothespins to hold on to it; they've hung weights from the end of it and worn wooden rings glued to the base. Onset comes as a result of fear—specifically, fear that such a thing might happen.)

Sex therapist Bernie Zilbergeld summarizes the situation with regard to temporary impotence in *The New Male Sexuality*: "Nonmedical erection problems are almost always due to one or more of the following: unrealistic expectations, lack of arousal, absence of the proper conditions, and the anxiety generated by the need for an erection. . . . If you are tense or anxious, if you are angry at your partner, if you aren't getting the physical and emotional stimulation you like, if you aren't turned on, if you are preoccupied with other matters—if any of these things are true, what makes you think you should have an erection? The answer, of course, is our sexual conditioning."

It's a man's thinking he *should* have an erection that causes performance anxiety—and maybe that's why some men have erections more easily when they shouldn't. As in the following joke: A man gets a prescription for Viagra from his doctor, who tells him to take one and then have sex with his wife within the hour. A little more than an hour later the man phones his doctor. "I've taken the Viagra but my wife isn't home," he says. "There's no one home but the maid."

The doctor says, "Then have sex with the maid."

"But, doctor," the man says, "I don't need Viagra to have sex with the maid."

PREVENTIVE MEDICINE FOR IMPOTENCE

Sex therapists used to be the ones in charge of erection problems—but now that the physiology is known, and it's clear erections are dependent on blood flow to the penis, MDs are in a position to give practical advice. Dr. Kaminetsky told me there were steps a man could take to stave off impotence, and they were the same as the steps you would take to prevent heart disease: Eat a healthy, low-fat diet, keep your weight, blood pressure and cholesterol down. Smoking is the worst thing for potency. Drinking isn't good, but it's not as bad as smoking. A man who uses too much cocaine may not be able to get an erection while he's under the influence of the drug.

Then there's bicycle-riding. One eminent Boston urologist, Dr. Irwin Goldstein, often comments during interviews on the link between impotence and bicycle-riding. Apparently the seat is the problem. On a narrow bike seat the cavernosal artery—which controls blood flow to the penis—is subjected to constant pounding. Men can avoid bike-related impotence by switching to a seat with oval openings in the saddle.

REMEDIES FOR IMPOTENCE

Traditionally, men with erection problems have tried to enhance their enthusiasm with aphrodisiacs. Mandrake root and other roots that resemble a penis have always been thought to have penis-invigorating properties. Certain animals have also been credited with magical sexual properties, because of the way they look, or behave. Rhino horn is particularly prized in the East, and the hunt for rhino horn to be ground up into sex tonics has made the rhino an endangered species.

Dogs, too, have had their day. In 1889 a distinguished French physiologist, Charles Brown-Sequard, then seventy-two years old, told an audience at the Société de Biologie in Paris that he had recently removed the testicles of a vigorous three-year-old dog, cut them in pieces, mashed them with water and injected himself with the filtrate. After ten years of abstinence, he said, he was once again potent and had just that morning had sex with his much younger wife. The announcement caused a sensation, but others who tried the experiment did not obtain the same results.

Thanks to modern technology we now have proven techniques for dealing with impotence, and no man needs to consider chopping up Fido to get relief.

PENIS IMPLANTS

Dr. Kaminetsky showed me a sample penis implant, the most effective permanent treatment for impotence. It was made of clear plastic and consisted of two thin tubes to be surgically inserted into the two erectile bodies in the penis, and a bulb called the reservoir that gets filled with saline solution and inserted behind the abdominal wall. A switching device is sewn into one of the testicles. ("Jack" described to me a similar device used by some female-to-male transsexuals.)

When the penis is at rest it's flaccid, but a bit stretched out. When a man wants to have sex he squeezes the wired testicle and the fluid in the reservoir fills up the cylinders, producing a nice erection. When sex is over, he presses the device in the scrotum again and the fluid drains back out. It sounds more like a physics experiment than a sex organ, but according to Dr. Kaminetsky it works quite well. It is a last resort, though, because it permanently destroys the erectile tissue.

Also, because a penis implant requires surgery, many couples decide against it. Dr. Kaminetsky described a typical scenario: "A man will come to see me who's impotent, and we'll go through all the things he might try and very often the woman he's with doesn't even know he's here. We'll talk about the penile implant and that's it; that's what he wants. He gets all excited. Then he comes back and says, 'My wife won't let me do it. She said, What are you, crazy?'"

"So what I do is I try to meet with the man and woman together, to explain to the woman that men view sex differently. Women view sex more as part of love, and they can have affection other ways. But if a man's not getting laid, if he can't fuck, he doesn't feel like a man. The woman feels guilty that the man's doing it for her when she doesn't care that much, or she's scared something's going to happen to him and it's going to be her fault. And I tell her, 'Your husband Mr. Jones loves you and he wants to have sex with you, but he's not doing this for you, he's doing this for himself, this is very important to him.'"

ERECTION DRUGS

The first anti-impotence drug, alprostadil, went on the market in 1995. Alprostadil, which goes under the trade names Muse, Caverject and Edex, is either injected into the base of the penis (Caverject, Edex) or inserted with an applicator into the tip of the penis (Muse), and it works by relaxing the smooth-muscle cells and opening up the arteries. In men for whom this drug is effective (over 50 percent of cases), erection comes on within five to twenty minutes; in fact, the man gets an erection whether he feels like it or not. An alprostadil erection can last an hour or more; in rare cases, particularly if the drug is being used recreationally by a man with normal arteries, it can cause a dangerously prolonged erection. A man with an erection more than four hours old is suffering from priapism and ought to visit a doctor for deflation. Eventually, a constant erection can lead to "wooden penis"; the penis becomes so fibrous from lack of oxygen that it can't get erections anymore. (Priapism may also be a side effect of sickle-cell anemia and certain tumors. It should always be attended to.)

VIAGRA: THE MALE PILL

By now most people who are interested in penises know about Viagra and related oral erection medications. A man takes a pill, and if it works for him he should have an erection within an hour or less. Men who were quoted in the media when Viagra first came out said the results were miraculous; they felt like teenagers again.

Viagra (generic name sildenafil) became an anti-impotence drug by accident. It was tested first as a drug to fight angina, the pain that comes from narrowing of the blood vessels near the heart. Though it wasn't effective against angina, test subjects wanted to keep their samples. The reason: The drug was giving them erections.

Viagra is said to be natural-feeling because it works with the chemicals released by the nervous system when a man is sexually aroused, and it won't be effective if he isn't aroused. There don't seem to be many side effects aside from an occasional flushed face, headache or upset stomach. Oh, yes, and 3 percent of men see everything with a slight bluish tinge, temporarily.

Viagra apparently has also been a factor in a number of deaths. The drug went on the market in April 1998, and by the end of November the FDA had received reports of 130 deaths that seemed to be Viagra-related. Viagra itself didn't kill anybody. Some Viagra users who had heart conditions probably died from the unusual exertion. Others may not have heeded the warnings. Viagra lowers blood pressure and shouldn't be taken with nitrates and other drugs that also lower blood pressure. (Those off-limits nitrates include amyl nitrate. Several men have died after taking Viagra and then getting high with poppers of amyl nitrate.)

Viagra's debut was an enormous success. By its third week on sale it had captured 94 percent of the impotence drug market, and doctors were writing forty thousand prescriptions a week. In its first three months, 2 million men were estimated to have tried it. Men began fine-tuning their dosage—100 mgs or 50, taken on a full or an empty stomach. Now that there was a cure, they didn't mind admitting in public that they might not always be rock-hard when they wanted to be. Even former senator Bob Dole admitted it. He said he'd had surgery for prostate cancer and later participated in the Viagra clinical trials, and he thought it was a great drug.

The advent of Viagra, a boon for men, has also been good for certain endangered species. Early in 1999 I heard a report that as a result of the availability of the impotence pill in the Far East, the trade in rhino horn and tiger penis had greatly diminished.

Viagra doesn't just give men their erections back, it changes the sexual equation. As soon as it came out, women began worrying in print about the effect on marriages and other long-term relationships. If old men could get it up again, they'd leave their wives for younger women. Younger men would start fooling around more. Why didn't they invent a pill to make guys considerate instead of potent? Men said they needed Viagra to regain the ground they'd lost to the women's movement. Philip Weiss of the *New York Observer* saw Viagra as an obvious baby boomers' drug. "They invented Viagra because their lives are too structured, they're in stuffy monogamous relationships and can't turn on. Forget all the window dressing—Viagra's not a gay drug, it's not a drug for women, it's not a drug for impotence. Viagra is the drug that is supposed to cure monogamy. Because monogamous sex is so . . . so, so fucking great."

On a more earnest note, articles here and there made the point that impotence was almost always a complex problem, part physical, part emotional. And that Viagra, which merely treated its physical aspects, could cause havoc in some relationships. Viagra was in that sense a stereotypical male solution. A man could take a pill and he wouldn't have to talk about it.

The fact is, though, that all of us are talking about it. For months after its launch there were new Viagra headlines every few days. Gradually, more related stories began cropping up in family newspapers, about everything from the structure of animal penises to the structure of penis-friendly bicycle seats. My friend Enrique thinks amassing information about penises and using it in conversation may be, like Viagra, a substitute in this age of sexually transmitted diseases for the former joys of promiscuity.

After many a long month's immersion in Penis World I still believe the more we know about them the better. No one's ever going to get bored with penises, because in the flesh each one is different—"just like snowflakes," I heard comedienne Margaret Cho say on TV. And as for the sanctity of the male mysteries, let's clear up the confusion. There are mysteries and then there are secrets.

Secrets aren't the same as mysteries, though they seem to be when they're hidden. Secrets can be told; mysteries just exist. The more we know about penises, the less we hide our feelings about them, the freer we can be with each other. Penises themselves are a mysterious and potent force, and they always will be, no matter what anyone says.

EPILOGUE

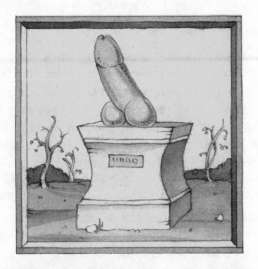

FAMOUS FOR
THEIR DICKS

The following is a compilation of stories about famous men and their penises. In case you're not really convinced about penis madness, consider this: There is no such subject as celebrity vaginas. No one ever wonders what a woman's vagina or clitoris looks like except in a sexual way; yet down deep most of us feel as if knowing the shape of a man's dick tells us something about his character. A famous man with a big penis proves that size equals power. A famous man whose penis is small has made himself powerful in order to compensate. A meek man with a big penis shows how weird life is.

EPILOGUE

HOLLYWOOD

There's always been gossip about movie star penises. Movie stars are the lovers everyone yearns for, and if they're ideal, of course their dicks should be big. But here's what movie star Betty Grable is reported to have said, in the 1940s: "They say the two best-hung men in Hollywood are Forrest Tucker and Milton Berle. What a shame—it's never the handsome ones. The bigger they are, the homelier."

Gary Griffin, in *Penis Enlargement Methods—Fact and Phallusy*, has a thirty-page section full of "well-endowed celebrities," half of it devoted to Hollywood. He gets his information from biographies, books of gossip and reports from readers who claim to have been intimate with celebrities. Of Griffin's Hollywood heavies I will list only the dead ones: Humphrey Bogart, Ward Bond, Jack Cassidy, Charlie Chaplin, Gary Cooper, Errol Flynn, Freddy Frank, Cary Grant, William Holden, Rock Hudson, John Ireland, John Loder, Dean Martin, Groucho Marx, Steve McQueen, Dennis O'Keefe, Walter Pidgeon, Aldo Ray, Frank Sinatra, Franchot Tone, Forrest Tucker.

MILTON BERLE

Milton Berle is such a consummate comedian that even the gossip about his penis seems like some kind of joke. In the 1950s, when he had his popular TV show, he called himself Uncle Miltie. He made funny noises, wore dresses and lipstick, did anything for a laugh, and hardly seemed to have a sex.

But all along, underneath his skirts, hung the most talked-about dick in Hollywood. In the musical *Out of*

This World, Cole Porter used Berle's dick in a lyric. The song is "Cherry Pies Ought to Be You." The goddess Juno and a Chicago gangster have had sex, and now they hate each other. When Juno sings, "Milton Berle ought to be you," she's casting aspersions on the size of the gangster's genitals.

Berle tells a funny story about his penis in his autobiography. He's in a locker room at a steam bath with a friend, and a friend of that friend. The man he hasn't met before begins razzing him about his reputation for having "a big one." Berle tries to discourage the man, but he's adamant. He wants to bet his is bigger than Berle's. Berle is beginning to get annoyed at this person he's just met when their mutual friend intercedes. "Go ahead, Milton," he says, "just take out enough to win."

ERROL FLYNN

Errol Flynn played swashbuckling rakes and seducers on-screen, and was also known to be one. A number of stories about him are penis stories, because he liked cock-centered practical jokes. He had such charm that his antics only added to his mystique.

One night he walked over to the house of his neighbor, the gossip columnist Hedda Hopper, and jerked off on her front door—and Hopper was amused.

Sometimes he took out his penis at a party and played the piano with it.

He used tight-fitting Australian swim shorts as underpants, and wore his cock pointing up, so you could see it peeking out of the waistband of his trousers.

"Such was his reputation," reported actor Iron Eyes Cody in his autobiography, "that I know of several perfectly sane directors . . . who actually asked to see it, right there on the set. . . . Errol would unzip and proceed to set the record straight. Regardless of who was present."

HUSBANDS OF ELIZABETH TAYLOR

Three husbands of Elizabeth Taylor, the so-called most beautiful woman in the world, are listed in Gary Griffin's *Penis Enlargement Methods* as "well-endowed celebrities"— Nicky Hilton, Eddie Fisher and John Warner. Either this is true, or people think it should be.

SPORTS

George Plimpton told me that when he was playing for the Detroit Lions, preparing to write his book *Paper Lion*, the players referred to really big penises as "knee-slappers." Plimpton said he was told that Roger Brown, a defensive tackle on the Lions in the 1960s, had a knee-slapper.

The most famous penis in sports—in terms of reported use—belongs to Wilt (the Stilt) Chamberlain. The 7 foot 1 inch Chamberlain, who retired from the Los Angeles Lakers in 1973, still holds the NBA record for most points scored in a game (100), most points scored in a season (4,029) and highest average number of points per game (50.4). In 1991 he staked his claim to another record, when he said in public that he'd had sex with more than 20,000 women. No other basketball superstar has publicly challenged this record—except for the flamboyant Dennis Rodman, who didn't say that he'd had more women, but rather that Wilt must have been lying about having so many. According to Gary Griffin, when he was coming close to retirement Wilt willingly displayed his penis at parties to women who inquired.

PENISES AS RELICS

DILLINGER

Given the association between penises, guns and macho behavior, it's only logical there would be a gangster with a famous penis. John Dillinger, public enemy number one during the 1930s, is that gangster. Many people believe Dillinger's dick was so enormous that it's been kept at the Smithsonian Institution, preserved in formaldehyde inside a glass jar.

At the Smithsonian they say they do not have any such thing. Nevertheless, every time the rumor is mentioned publicly people start writing the Smithsonian, wanting to know if it's true, and what are the dick's dimensions, and how can they see it, or get a photograph. The Dillinger's penis rumor is a joke around the Smithsonian, but an annoying kind of joke, since it comes up so often.

My source at the Smithsonian said the story about the size of Dillinger's penis probably started when his dead body was stretched out on a cot, under a sheet, and there seemed to be a bulge at its midsection. The story about its being severed and ending up in a jar may have originated at the time when the Army Medical Museum was on the mall near the Smithsonian. That museum, now housed at Walter Reed Hospital, also never had Dillinger's penis. But it does contain some other truly marvelous oddities, including a kind of Siamese twin penis that has one stem with two heads.

NAPOLEON

Officially Napoleon was said to have died of stomach cancer while in exile on St. Helena. But some authorities believe he was actually poisoned with small doses of arsenic. When he died he was fat and practically hairless, two symptoms of slow arsenic poisoning. Also, his sex organs were said to be extremely small, and it's implied the arsenic must have shrunk them. After all, a great French leader, famous in his youth for his sexual escapades, could hardly have been afflicted with micropenis.

When I first started working on this book, I heard about Dr. John Lattimer, former chair of the urology department at Columbia Presbyterian hospital in New York, who was said to own Napoleon's penis. I wrote to Dr. Lattimer asking to see the relic and to interview him about the correlations, if any, between a man's penis and his character. I got no answer, and when I spoke with his assistant on the telephone she told me the doctor had nothing to say.

"Can you just tell me whether he actually owns the penis?" I asked her.

She said, "I told you, he doesn't want to talk about it."

It seemed strange to me that a person who'd gone to the expense and trouble of buying Napoleon's penis wouldn't want to talk about it. What else is it, if not a conversation piece? Then again, any conversation can grow tiresome if repeated too many times.

Some months later, the writer Brendan Gill told me his Napoleon's penis story. "Once in the early 1960s I visited a very distinguished bibliophile and her lawyer husband, also a great bibliophile. She was showing me around the library and she said to me, 'Oh, by the way, would you care to see Napoleon's penis?'

"I said, 'My God, you of all people—how in the world did you acquire that?'

"She said, 'We bought it at an odd-lot sale, and among the odd lot was this penis.'"

She pointed to the box it was in, but he declined, and she didn't press him. It sounds as if the object was losing its charm for her. "She said, 'It's just as well. It's more of a tendon than anything else by now.'"

A few years later the couple put the penis up for auction. Napoleon's penis was sold at Christie's in 1968. In 1977 it was auctioned again in Paris; a private buyer got it for 7,000 francs. Early in 1999 *New York* magazine ran a story about Dr. Lattimer and his collection of "keepsakes from history's darker moments." Therein, Dr. Lattimer admitted he owned Napoleon's penis, having bought it from dealers in Paris seven years earlier. A Napoleon expert quoted by *New York* doubted its authenticity—over the years, he said, two different people had offered to sell Napoleon's penis to him.

Brendan Gill, who got around a lot, also told me he'd seen a table at Biltmore, the Vanderbilt estate in North Carolina, with a sign on it that said, "In the drawer of this table once resided Napoleon's heart."

RASPUTIN

Grigory Rasputin, who became the most trusted advisor to Nicholas and Alexandra of Russia, was a master seducer. He had hypnotic eyes, and promoted himself as a clairvoyant and a miraculous healer. So persuasive was he that many of his followers believed he was Christ reincarnated. Those who were against him called him the Holy Devil.

Even his daughter Maria said he conducted his religious rites as if they were orgies, and in this enterprise, if she's to be trusted as a witness, he was aided by the Almighty, who had endowed him with a very big dick. Here's a description from Maria Rasputin's biography of her father:

"Mention has been made of the Shiva lingam and other phallic symbols, and the way they were worshiped as the

215

representations of the creative principle. When his female devotees danced their dervishlike dances around his nude figure, they, too, were drawn to the worship of his phallus, endowing it with mystical qualities as well as sexual ones, for it was an extraordinary member indeed, measuring a good thirteen inches when fully erect. Theirs was by no means a wholly lustful approach at the start of the rite, but a worship of God in His Priapean form; and whichever of the female disciples was the first to perform fellatio upon him did so in a sense of religious practice. Of course, as their passions were aroused, there was a tendency to forget the ritualistic aspect of the ceremony, and the participants would fall into a general orgy, seeking whatever outlet for their lusts was available."

Rasputin was murdered by Prince Felix Yussupov, who wrote about it himself. It was 1916; Yussupov and co-conspirators feared Rasputin's power over the Czar and were afraid the monk was a spy for Germany, with which Russia was at war. The prince invited the monk to tea. He fed him cream cakes and wine laced with potassium cyanide. The monk ate and drank and went on talking. The prince shot the monk and still he didn't die. He was shot again and raped and castrated and finally thrown in the ice-covered Neva River. He died not from any of the gunshot wounds or the poison, but by drowning.

Regarding the penis factor, there are many questions that could be asked—was Rasputin powerful because his dick was so big, did his dick just seem big because he was powerful, and so on. It's hard to distinguish fact from legend in this case, but I can report that Patte Barham, Maria Rasputin's coauthor, claims she actually saw the thing, in 1968 when the biography was being written. It reposed, Barham says, in the apartment of an old and ailing Russian peasant woman in Paris, lying on velvet inside a polished wooden box on a bureau beneath Rasputin's picture. It looked like a foot-long, blackened, overripe banana.

FAMOUS USES OF PENIS SKIN

If penises are magical, then objects covered in penis skin will also have magic—unless you think that skinning someone's penis is a revolting barbarism. Enrique told me that when he was a child in Venezuela someone showed him a beautiful eighteenth-century knife, with a shiny blade and a black leather handle. This handle, he was told, was made from the skin of the penis of a black slave. The black man's penis was meant to endow the knife with power.

Usually, when men want to make things out of penis skin, they choose the penises of mammals, whales in particular. If any penis is going to have magical powers, a whale penis will. A whale erection is one foot wide and ten feet long—that's taller than any known human being.

In Melville's *Moby Dick* there's a description of the way whale blubber is sliced up. The mincer, the man in charge, dresses himself for the task in a three-foot-long section of the dried pelt of the whale's penis, so he seems to be wearing a cassock. As for whale sperm, the narrator Ishmael, who's put to work squeezing the lumps out of it, thinks it's heavenly: "Such a cleaner! such a sweetener! such a softener! such a delicious mollifier! After having my hands in it for only a few minutes, my fingers felt like eels. . . . While bathing in that bath, I felt divinely free from all ill-will, or petulance, or malice, of any sort whatsoever."

Aristotle Onassis, on his yacht, *Christina,* had bar stools covered with whale-penis skin. He liked to be able to inform a guest she was sitting on the biggest dick in the world.

217

FISH AND ANIMALS
WITH NOTABLE PENISES

PIGS

A boar has a slender penis, about eighteen inches long, with a thin corkscrew tip. A sow has ridges on her cervix to accommodate the shape of the boar. When they have sex the boar thrusts and thrusts until his corkscrew tip is firmly locked into the sow's cervical ridges. Then he ejaculates, a pint of semen at a time.

SHARKS

In most shark species the males have two long, tapering penises jutting out from their undersides. These penises are called "claspers," although they do not clasp. Their tips are fanlike, equipped to spray when the male ejaculates. A male shark copulates upside down and he may use one or both claspers to do the deed. Because sharks are so dangerous, many details of their sex lives are not known.

OPOSSUMS

An opossum penis is forked, to accommodate the double organs of the female opossum. His prick seems to be in one piece when the male opossum urinates, but when he's ready for sex and his foreskin retracts, his penis splits in two.

HORSES

Horse dicks become erect when they fill with blood, like human dicks. But a horse has more control than a man and sometimes when he's not having an erection he likes to let his long dick just hang out. Because of this habit many people have seen horse dicks; hence the expression, "hung like a horse." Stallions keep harems and are obsessed with mares; however, their version of the sex act is over in no time.

ELEPHANTS

An elephant penis is four to five feet long and S-shaped when erect, with an enormous bulb at the end. When a male elephant has an erection standing upwind of a female, the female can smell it. During the few days that the female is receptive, elephant couples make the most of it, copulating several times each day. Pregnancy lasts another two years.

FLATWORMS

Flatworms are hermaphrodites. They all have small, pointed penises, shaped like the tips of ballpoint pens. When two flatworms meet and want to mate, a penis fencing match ensues, and what they're fighting over is who gets to be the male. The one who wins penetrates the other one's flesh with his penis, discharging sperm and remaining free to fence again. The other becomes female and pregnant.

ORIENTAL COCKROACHES

According to an article in the *New York Times*, the penis of an oriental cockroach unfolds, "blade by blade, like a Swiss Army knife."

FAMOUS POP CULTURE PENISES

JOE CAMEL

Joe Camel, the cartoon camel used to advertise Camel cigarettes, was so popular with teenagers that eventually he was banned from Camel ads. The reason for his popularity was phallic; if you turned him upside down his nose looked like a penis penetrating a vagina.

THE LITTLE MERMAID

On the original cover of the video for the Disney animated film *The Little Mermaid*, one of the turrets of the castle is shaped like a penis. All teenagers know this and the video is popular partly for its cover.

THE LITTLE MERMAID, II

During the wedding scene in *The Little Mermaid*, the clergyman appears to have a hard-on, though Disney denies that he does. This scene is a hit with teenagers but not with the Southern Baptist Convention.

HOWARD STERN

Howard Stern, the outspoken radio and TV personality, is as responsible as anybody for popularizing penis talk in the 1990s. People find his penis talk acceptable, or even endearing, because he keeps saying how small his own dick is. Here's a passage from his autobiography, *Private Parts*: "Having a small penis has haunted me throughout my life. Whenever I'm with a bunch of guys, like going to Atlantic City to gamble or stuff, and we have to make a stop on the way to urinate, I always make a beeline for the stalls. I can't do it at a urinal. God forbid someone should see my puny pecker. I barely clear the zipper. If all the stalls are filled and I *have* to use a urinal, I press up so close to it that it's like I'm humping the porcelain."

Anyone who's insecure about anything can feel close to Howard. With his credentials he also gets full permission to talk about other guys' dicks.

By the way, Howard's wife Alison is quoted in *Private Parts* as saying Howard's penis size is "fine."

U.S. PRESIDENTS

Although John F. Kennedy was known to have had a hyperactive sex life in the White House, it was his vice president and successor, Lyndon Baines Johnson, who was the phallic one. When he was in college he loved to show off his dick, according to one Internet trivia quiz, and his pet name for it was Jumbo. As President, he often gave Jumbo an airing. For one thing, he used his bathroom as an adjunct to his office; he continued to conduct business there while he was relieving himself. Also, it was said reporters had to swim naked with him in the White House pool if they wanted to get their stories.

When he was running for office he was said to say things like, "Gentlemen, I have a hard-on for the presidency"; and when he got there, things like, "I don't trust a man until I have his pecker in my pocket." Once when some reporters were pestering him about why we were in Vietnam he became exasperated, unzipped his fly, pulled out his dick and said, "This is why."

A famous story from his presidency had it that a woman on his staff, while staying at the Johnson Ranch to do some work, woke up one night to feel someone in bed with her. Then she heard Johnson say, "Move over, honey, it's your president."

Stories like this made Johnson sound like someone who thought he could get away with anything and who, therefore, could. They added to his image as an earthy and powerful man.

In the late 1990s stories circulated about Bill Clinton's

penis, but they didn't particularly add to his image. We knew about the penis because, it was said, he'd been indiscreet about where he put it. Paula Jones, when she was suing the President for sexual harassment, claimed for a long time that she could prove her case by describing his penis, and eventually we found out what she said she'd seen: It was about five inches long when erect, as big around as a quarter, and bent. This sounds respectable enough, but not what you would call presidential.

For a few days in the newspapers there was speculation that if Jones was telling the truth the President might suffer from Peyronies disease. Men with this condition— which may either be genetic or develop after some trauma to the penis, usually during sex—have plaque or scar tissue in their penises that causes them to bend to one side. In severe cases a penis with Peyronies disease can end up looking like a pretzel. (The Byzantine emperor Heraclius —who reigned from 610–641 A.D., took back the empire from the invading Persians and rescued a fragment of the true cross—must have suffered from Peyronies disease. At the end of his life his penis was said to bend straight up, so that when he urinated he had to be careful not to squirt himself in the eye.) After the first talk about President Clinton's possible Peyronies disease, gossips started saying he'd had surgery to correct his condition. Then the matter was dropped.

Truman Capote, a notoriously engaging liar, claimed in the Capote biography by Gerald Clarke that he saw all the Kennedys naked and that they, too, were not exactly presidential. "What I don't understand is why everybody said the Kennedys were so sexy. I know a lot about cocks —I've seen an awful lot of them—and if you put all the Kennedys together, you wouldn't have one good one. I used to see Jack when I was staying with Loel and Gloria

Guinness in Palm Beach. I had a little guest cottage with its own private beach, and he would come down so he could swim in the nude. He had absolutely nuthin'! Bobby was the same way; I don't know how he had all those children. As for Teddy—forget it."

WRITERS AND THEIR PENISES

Stories of writers and their penises have a melancholy cast.

GUY DE MAUPASSANT

In Frank Harris's fat and sexually explicit autobiography, *My Life and Loves*, most of the sex stories are about himself. But he makes an exception for the great French story writer Guy de Maupassant, whose sexual prowess he can't help but envy at first. When Maupassant was in his thirties, Harris says, he could still ejaculate six times in a night and make love twenty times. ("After the sixth there's no more semen, so why not?") He could have an erection at will (Harris thought he himself was the only man who could do that). But Maupassant was reckless with his passions, and because of his extraordinary powers, women were his downfall. Physically he couldn't take so much lovemaking. His last, frenzied affair, with a married woman, finally drove him into the madhouse (syphilis may have helped). He died there, aged forty-three.

FRANZ KAFKA

In Alan Bennett's comedy *Kafka's Dick*, the ghost of Kafka, and the ghost of Kafka's father, and the ghost of his biographer and publisher Max Brod, visit a suburban English couple, Linda and Sydney. Sydney is a Kafka expert, writing an article. Hermann Kafka has come to set the record straight. Everyone thinks he was a terrible father, he says, but actually he was great. He blackmails Franz into going along with the deception. Franz will say anything to keep his own most shameful secret. But it comes out anyway. The joke is on him—his dick is only three inches long.

HENRY JAMES

Leon Edel, in his massive biography, considers the possibility that Henry James's penis may have been wounded when he was a young man. James often spoke of a mysterious wound he received while helping to put out a fire. He said the wound was painful and embarrassing yet not at all dangerous. In the end Edel concludes that James would not have been able to joke about eunuchs, as he sometimes did, if he were one himself. But some sort of castration might explain James's lifelong—as far as anyone knows—celibacy. And also his awfully hesitant and orotund prose style and his refusal to get to the point. Or, as Will Self puts it in *Cock & Bull*, "Since poor Henters couldn't fuck anybody else, he resolved to fuck us all up with his serpentine sentences . . . uncoiling inside our minds like ever-lengthening weenies."

F. SCOTT FITZGERALD

Fitzgerald's story is a perfect example of the way a man can be spooked about his penis. As Ernest Hemingway tells it in *A Moveable Feast*, the subject comes up after a lunch in a Paris restaurant. "You know," Fitzgerald says, referring to his wife, "I never slept with anyone except Zelda."

"No, I didn't."

"I thought I had told you."

"No. You told me a lot of things but not that."

"That is what I have to ask you about."

"Good. Go on."

"Zelda said that the way I was built I could never make any woman happy and that was what upset her originally. She said it was a matter of measurements. I have never felt the same since she said that and I have to know truly."

Hemingway takes Fitzgerald to the men's room and has a look. "You're perfectly fine," he says, but Fitzgerald isn't convinced. Hemingway takes Fitzgerald to the Louvre to look at some statues and compare them with himself but after the viewing Fitzgerald is still doubtful. Hemingway gives him advice about sexual technique, using a pillow to change the angle of penetration and so on. Fitzgerald says there's a woman he's interested in but he's afraid to have an affair because of what Zelda said about his size. Hemingway tells him that's why Zelda said it.

FAMOUS FOR THEIR DICKS ALONE

JOHN WAYNE BOBBITT

John Wayne Bobbitt is our ultimate dickhead, and he's made this condition work for him. When his wife amputated his penis and it was sewn back on, he capitalized on the one special thing about himself, and began exhibiting it. Barely a year after his reattachment surgery he released his first semiautobiographical X-rated video, *John Wayne Bobbitt . . . Uncut.*

Bobbitt plays himself, an actress plays Lorena. Lorena gets mad when he comes to bed one night—after a boys' night out at a topless bar—because first he fondles her breasts and wakes her up, then it turns out he's too drunk

225

for sex. Every woman in the audience knows how infuriating his behavior is, but John hasn't got a clue. Unfortunately, Lorena is also a bit dense. She begs and begs him to get hard, as if begging would do the trick. When he just won't listen, she takes a knife and slices his dick off, gets in the car with it, drives for a while and throws it out the window.

When next we see John his dick has been retrieved and he's in the hospital, recovering from surgery. It's the beginning of his new life. As he says, "Ever since this whole thing started, all everyone ever wants to see is my penis." The first to be so curious are the nurses—they look at it, they get excited, so does he. He'd been told he wouldn't be able to use the dick for sex for maybe two years, but in fact it's working just fine already. Or sort of. The only interesting thing in the rest of the video, which follows Bobbitt's fortunes as a sex object, is the sight of his poor, put-upon dick, size low-average with a ridge around the middle where it was reattached, struggling to get the call to action from his brain.

He's since made a second film, *Frankenpenis*, about how he had penis enlargement surgery and the job was botched.

PORFIRIO RUBIROSA

Rubirosa was an emissary in the service of the Dominican Republic who flourished during the 1940s and '50s, and counted among his five wives the two most famous American heiresses of his generation, Doris Duke and Barbara Hutton. His conquests were innumerable. "While he was incapable of being true to any one woman, he was devoted to any woman who could afford him," says one of Duke's biographers. He was dapper, swarthy and charming, and he knew how to pay attention to a woman. He also had a penis of true distinction. It's described in *Too Rich: The Family Secrets of Doris Duke* as more than eleven inches long, with a six-inch circumference—"much like the last foot of a Louisville Slugger baseball bat with the consistency of a not completely inflated volley ball."

But size isn't everything, and Rubirosa was famous because he cultivated his gift. One of his nicknames was "Rubirosa the Hosa." Another was "Toujours Pret," meaning Always Ready.

"His purpose was to satisfy women," Duke once said. ". . . his prick was so large that it seemed to be in a state of eternal erection. I don't think that he really felt anything when he was making love but he was able to do whatever I wanted for endless hours. I was always the focus during sex. All that mattered was that I be satisfied. He simply wanted to make every woman on earth experience the ultimate climax."

Barbara Hutton wrote in her notebooks, "His lovemaking secret is that he practices an Egyptian technique called Imsak. No matter how aroused he becomes, he doesn't allow himself to complete the act. What he enjoys about it is the sense of control, beyond the threshold. His pleasure derives from totally arousing his partner while he remains aloof, the absolute master of the situation."

Doris Duke said Rubirosa, to please her, even sometimes faked an orgasm.

If anyone deserves the epithet "cocksman," he does. So well-known was he in his prime that in the finest European restaurants when people wanted the waiter to bring the big pepper mill to the table, they asked him for the "Rubirosa."

THE BOOK OF
THE PENIS:
RESOURCES

MAGAZINES:

INCHES
Mavety Media Group, Ltd.
462 Broadway, 4th floor
New York, NY 10013

PFIQ (Piercing *Fans International Quarterly*)
Editorial: Gauntlet, Inc.
537 Castro Street
San Francisco, CA 94114–2511
(415) 552–0505
fax: (415) 552–0874
e-mail: jimward@gauntlet.com

Subscriptions & back issues:
Gauntlet Customer Service
2215–R Market Street
Box 801
San Francisco, CA 94114
(800) RINGS-2-U
(#46 and #48 feature pierced penises)

PENIS RESOURCES

MEN'S HEALTH
Rodale Press, Inc.
33 East Minor Street
Emmaus, PA 18098
(610) 967–5171
www.menshealth.com

ART IN AMERICA
575 Broadway
New York, NY 10012
(212) 941–2800

CLUBS:

SMALL, ETC.
J. Meisler
P.O. Box 610294
Bayside, NY 11361–0294
web site: http://www.trweb.com/small

WEB SITES:

SIZE
Definitive Penis Size Survey:
   http://www.connection.com/~dickie/
Complete Kinsey measurement statistics:
   http://www.drcanada.com/stats.htm
Vacuum Pumpers Site:
   http://207.211.39.119/pump/index.htm
Vacuum Pumpers Forum:
   http://207.211.39.119/pumpforum3/wwwboard3.html

CIRCUMCISION & UNCIRCUMCISION
Circumcision Information and Resource Page:
  http://www.cirp.org/
Circumcision/Foreskin Restoration Resource Page:
  http://www.4skin.com/restore/niks4wen
Chymmylt Foreskin Restoration Site (includes clear color
photos of circumcised, uncircumcised and restored foreskin penises; also includes links to information about infant circumcision):
  http://www.4skin.com/chymmylt/frames.html
Foreskin Restoration Male Sexuality:
  http://net.indra.com/~shredder/restore/index.html

PIERCING
Body Piercing and Modification Forum:
  http://207.211.39.119/pumpforum9/wwwboard9.html

MASTURBATION
JackinWorld:
  http://www.jackinworld.com/home.html
Masturbation Home Page:
  http://www.masturbationpage.com

GARY GRIFFIN BOOKS
Added Dimensions publishing:
  http://www.male.com/index.shtml

TATTOOISTS:

Dmitri at Kaleidoscope
365 Canal Street
New York, NY 10013
(212) 274–8006

PENIS RESOURCES

Mad Dog at Mad Dog Tattoo
(415) 552–1297
www.maddogtattoo.com
(web site includes a gallery of beautiful—nonphallic—
tattoos, and a monthly feature on "moments in the history
of gay tattooing.") e-mail: maddog@maddogtattoo.com

PIERCERS:

Gauntlet
144 Fifth Avenue
New York, NY 10011
(212) 229–0180
www.gauntlet.com

ART GALLERIES:

GAY ART
Leslie-Lohman Gay Art Foundation
127 Prince Street, basement
New York, NY 10012

SURREALISTS
Ubu Gallery
16 East 78th Street
New York, NY 10021
(212) 794–4444

SEX TOYS:

The Leather Man, Inc.
111 Christopher Street
New York, NY 10014
(212) 243–5339

Good Vibrations
1210 Valencia Street
San Francisco, CA 94110
(415) 974–8980
www.goodvibes.com (web site is friendly and informative about its products, and stores in San Francisco and Berkeley host after-hours events.)

SELECTED BIBLIOGRAPHY

The Holy Bible: Revised Standard Version. New York: Meridian, 1962.

Anand, Margo. *The Art of Sexual Ecstasy*. New York: Tarcher/ G. P. Putnam's Sons, 1989.

Anderson, Dan and Berman, Maggie. *Sex Tips for Straight Women from a Gay Man*. New York: Regan Books/HarperCollins, 1997.

An Old Practitioner. *The Secret Sins of Society or Philosophy of the Sexes*. Chicago: Lake City Publishing Co., 1882.

Banner, Lois. "The Fashionable Sex, 1100–1600." *History Today*, April 1992.

Bennett, Alan. *Kafka's Dick*. New York: Samuel French, Inc., 1986.

Bentley, Richard. *Erotic Art*. New York: Gallery Books, 1984.

Berle, Milton, with Frankel, Haskell. *Milton Berle*. New York: Delacorte Press, 1974.

Bettelheim, Bruno. *Symbolic Wounds*. Glencoe, IL: The Free Press, 1954.

Bigelow, Jim, Ph.D. *The Joy of Uncircumcising*. Aptos, CA: Hourglass Book Publishing, 1995.

Blackburn, Julia. *The Emperor's Last Island*. New York: Vintage, 1991.

Brown, Donald E., Edwards, James W. and Moore, Ruth P. *The Penis Inserts of Southeast Asia*. Berkeley, CA: Center for South and Southeast Asia Studies, University of California at Berkeley, 1988.

Bryk, Felix. *Dark Rapture,* trans. Dr. Arthur J. Norton. New York: Walden Publications, 1939.

SELECTED BIBLIOGRAPHY

Castleman, Michael. *Sexual Solutions*. New York: Touchstone/ Simon & Schuster, 1989.

Chia, Mantak and Arava, Douglas Abrams. *The Multi-Orgasmic Man*. San Francisco: HarperCollins, 1996.

Clarke, Gerald. *Capote*. New York: Simon & Schuster, 1988.

Danielou, Alain. *Gods of Love and Ecstasy*. Rochester, VT: Inner Traditions, 1982.

————. *The Phallus,* trans. Jon Graham. Rochester, VT: Inner Traditions, 1995.

De Marley, Diana. *Fashion for Men*. New York: Holmes and Meier, 1985.

Diamond, Jared. "The Best Ways to Sell Sex." *Discover,* May 1996.

Douglas, Nik and Slinger, Penny. *The Alchemy of Ecstasy*. Rochester, VT: Destiny Books, 1979.

Duke, Pony and Thomas, Jason. *Too Rich*. New York: Harper-Collins, 1996.

Forshufvud, Sten. *Who Killed Napoleon?* trans. Alan Houghton Brodrick. London: Hutchinson, 1961.

Freud, Sigmund. *Introductory Lectures on Psycho-Analysis* (1920), trans. and ed. James Strachey. New York: Liveright/W. W. Norton & Company, 1966.

————. *New Introductory Lectures on Psycho-Analysis* (1933), trans. and ed. James Strachey. New York: W. W. Norton & Company, 1965.

Graves, Robert. *The Greek Myths: 1*. London: Penguin Books, 1960.

Griffin, Gary. *Penis Enlargement Methods—Fact & Phallusy*, 9th edition. Palm Springs, CA: Added Dimensions Publishing, 1996.

Harris, Frank. *My Life and Loves* (1925), ed. John F. Gallagher. New York: Grove Press, 1963.

Hemingway, Ernest. *A Moveable Feast* (1964). New York: Touchstone, 1992.

SELECTED BIBLIOGRAPHY

Heymann, C. David. *Poor Little Rich Girl*. New York: Random House, 1984.

Higham, Charles. *Errol Flynn*. New York: Doubleday, 1980.

Hite, Shere. *The Hite Report on Male Sexuality*. New York: Ballantine Books, 1981.

Hollander, Anne. *Sex and Suits*. New York: Kodansha, 1994.

Hooven, F. Valentine III. *Tom of Finland*. New York: St. Martin's Press, 1993.

Hopkins, Jerry and Sugerman, Danny. *No One Here Gets Out Alive*. New York: Warner Books, 1980.

Huntingford, G. W. B. *The Galla of Ethiopia and the Kingdoms of Kafa and Janjero*. London: International African Institute, 1955.

Keuls, Eva C. *The Reign of the Phallus*. Berkeley, CA: University of California Press, 1985.

Kinsey, Alfred C., Pomeroy, Wardell B. and Martin, Clyde E. *Sexual Behavior in the Human Male*. Philadelphia: W.B. Saunders Co., 1948.

Knight, Richard Payne. *A Discourse on the Worship of Priapus* (1786) and Wright, Thomas. *The Worship of the Generative Powers* (1866), reprinted in *Sexual Symbolism*. New York: Julian Press, 1957.

Lawrence, D. H. *Lady Chatterley's Lover* (1928). New York: Pocket Books, Inc., 1959.

Lawrenson, Helen. "How Now, Fellatio! Why Dost Thou Tarry?" *Esquire*, May 1977.

Levins, Hoag. *American Sex Machines*. Holbrook, MA: Adams Media Corporation, 1996.

Love, Brenda. *Encyclopedia of Unusual Sex Practices*. Fort Lee, NJ: Barricade Books, 1992.

Mailer, Norman. *Advertisements for Myself*. London: Flamingo, 1961.

Mansfield, Stephanie. *The Richest Girl in the World*. New York: G. P. Putnam's Sons, 1992.

SELECTED BIBLIOGRAPHY

Melville, Herman. *Moby Dick* (1851). New York: Signet Classics, 1961.

Miller, Merle. *Lyndon*. New York: G. P. Putnam's Sons, 1980.

Molinier, Pierre. Winnipeg, Canada: Plug In Editions/Santa Monica, CA: Smart Art Press, undated.

Morrisroe, Patricia. *Mapplethorpe*. New York: Random House, 1995.

Parsons, Alexandra. *Facts & Phalluses*. New York: St. Martin's Press, 1989.

Rabelais, François. *The Histories of Gargantua and Pantagruel*, trans. J. M. Cohen. London: Penguin Books, 1955.

Rasputin, Maria and Barham, Patte. *Rasputin*. Englewood Cliffs, NJ: Prentice-Hall, 1977.

Rawson, Hugh. *Wicked Words*. New York: Crown Publishers, 1989.

———. *A Dictionary of Euphemisms & Other Doubletalk*. New York: Crown Publishers, 1981.

Remondino, Peter Charles. *History of Circumcision, From the Earliest Times to the Present*. New York: AMS Press, 1974.

Rice, Edward. *Captain Sir Richard Francis Burton*. New York: Charles Scribner's Sons, 1990.

Richie, Donald and Ito, Kenkichi. *The Erotic Gods*. Tokyo: Zulushinsha, 1967.

Ridley, Matt. *The Red Queen*. New York: Penguin Books, 1993.

Roth, Philip. *Portnoy's Complaint* (1967). New York: Vintage, 1994.

Rout, Kathleen. *Eldridge Cleaver*. Boston: Wayne Publishers, 1991.

Schloss, Marc R. *The Hatchet's Blood*. Tucson, AZ: University of Arizona Press, 1988.

Schwartz, Kit. *The Male Member*. New York: St. Martin's Press, 1985.

SELECTED BIBLIOGRAPHY

Scott, George Riley. *Phallic Worship*. London: Senate, 1966.

Self, Will. *Cock & Bull*. New York: Vintage, 1992.

Silver, Burton and Busch, Heather. *Kokigami*. Berkeley, CA: Ten Speed Press, 1990.

Simons, G. L. *The Phallic Mystique*. New York: Pinnacle Books, 1973.

Steinberg, Leo. *The Sexuality of Christ in Renaissance Art and in Modern Oblivion*. New York: Pantheon 1983.

Stern, Howard. *Private Parts*. New York: Pocket Books, 1994.

Stone, Lee Alexander. *The Story of Phallicism* (1927). New York: AMS Press, 1976.

Strage, Mark. *The Durable Fig Leaf*. New York: William Morrow, 1980.

Strong, Bryan and DeVault, Christine. *Human Sexuality*. Mountain View, CA: Mayfield Publishing Company, 1994.

Styrsky, Jindrich. *Emilie Comes to Me in a Dream* (1933). New York: Ubu Gallery, 1997.

Tannahill, Reay. *Sex in History*. New York: Stein and Day, 1980.

Taylor, G. Rattray. *Sex in History*. New York: Vanguard Press, 1970.

Thorn, Mark. *Taboo No More*. New York: Shapolsky Publishers, 1990.

Ucko, Peter J. "Penis Sheaths: A Comparative Study." Proceedings of the Royal Anthropological Institute of Great Britain and Ireland for 1969.

Vale, V. and Juno, Andrea, eds. *Modern Primitives*. San Francisco: Re/Search Publications, 1989.

Vatsyayana. *The Kama Sutra*, trans. Sir Richard Burton and R. R. Arbuthnot; ed. W. G. Archer. New York: Capricorn Books, 1963.

Vonnegut, Kurt. *Breakfast of Champions*. New York: Delacorte Press/Seymour Lawrence, 1973.

SELECTED BIBLIOGRAPHY

Wallace, Robert A. *How They Do It*, New York: Morrow Quill Paperbacks, 1980.

Walters, Margaret. *The Nude Male*. New York and London: Paddington Press, Ltd., 1978.

Weiermair, Peter. *Wilhelm von Gloeden*. Köln: Taschen, 1996.

Zilbergeld, Bernie, Ph.D. *The New Male Sexuality*. New York: Bantam Books, 1992.

ACKNOWLEDGMENTS

This book could not have been researched and written without the generous assistance of my friends and acquaintances and the people with penis information to whom they introduced me. I'm grateful to everyone who gave me moral support, told me stories, lent me books, submitted to my questioning and otherwise helped me explore the subject. Thanks in particular to all who are mentioned in the text and to those, below, who aren't:

Cynthia Adler, John Ash, Betsy Baker, Tina Barney, Mike Berg, Marilyn Berkman, April Bernard, Jeffrey Bishop, Laurel Blossom, Beth Bosworth, Tom Breidenbach, Kathy Brew, Kitty Brewster, Michael Brownstein, Gerald Busby, Frederick Ted Castle, Gary Clevidence, Bill Cole, Williams Cole, Janet Coleman, J. C. Compton, Barbara Ellmann, Kathleen Gallander, Morris Golde, Michele Goodhue, Liz Grace, Scott Griffin, Anthony Haden-Guest, Judy Halevi, Griffin Hausbury, James Holmes, Ann Hoyt, Alexandra Isles, Alfred Jaretzki, M.D., Ann Kaupp, Brad Kessler, Willa Kim, Jill Krementz, Carol Lee, M.D., Marianne Macy, Jaime Manrique, Maxine Margolis, Harry Mathews, Julia A. Mayo, Ph.D., Eugene Meyers, Jerald T. Mlanich, Ted Mooney, Michael Moore, Raimundo Mora, Richd C. Neuweiler, Darragh Park, Andrea Purcigliotti, Jane Roberts, Stephanie Rose, Hugh Seidman, Harvey Shapiro, Colleen Sharp, Michael Shulan, Milton Simpson, Dustin Smith, Stephanie Smolinsky, Jennifer Sokolov, Bill Sullivan, Leonard Todd, John Wells, Susan Wheeler, David Zakin, M.D.

Special thanks to my special consultants, Roberto Guerra and Richard Osterweil.

ACKNOWLEDGMENTS

Thanks to Adam Boxer and Rosa Esman of the Ubu Gallery, Sal Monetti of the Leslie-Lohman Gay Art Foundation, Amy Levine of the SEICUS Library, Hesh Samalkar of the Asia Society.

Thanks to those whose professional guidance helped the book take shape: Ira Silverberg, Anton Mueller, Amy Hundley and Morgan Entrekin at Grove Press, and my agent, Jane Gelfman. And thanks to a perfect design team: Chip Kidd, Sergio Ruzzier and Charles Rue Woods, art director and copywriter extraordinaire.